STAY ON TARGET

Build Muscle, Lose Fat, and Get the Motivation to Succeed Using a Military-Proven Nutrition and Exercise Plan Anyone Can Do

BY: CHRIS LEHTO

www.ChrisLehto.com

To receive free guides, as well as updates on my future books, join my readers list at: www.chrislehto.com.

Copyright © 2016 Chris Lehto

Publishing services provided by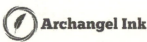

ISBN: 1515163725
ISBN-13: 978-1515163725

Table of Contents

PART 1: MINDSET 1

Chapter 1: Your Brain Has Its Own Agenda 3

Chapter 2: *Star Wars* Is Better than *Top Gun* 13

Chapter 3: True Change is Long-Term 21

PART 2: WORKOUT 31

Chapter 4: Task 1: Start, Maintain, and Track a Training Program ... 33

Chapter 5: Workout Targets 41

Chapter 6: Workout Threats 49

Chapter 7: Workout Program 57

    Two 4-day programs for the gym 60

    Two 4-Day programs for body weight exercises 62

Chapter 8: Minimize Time over Target with 4 Tactics 67

Chapter 9: Avoid (or Suppress) the Threats and Hit the Targets 77

PART 3: NUTRITION 89

Chapter 10: Task 2: Start, Maintain, and Track a
Food Plan.. 91

Chapter 11: Our 100-Year-Old Calorie System Is
Incorrect... 97

Chapter 12: Nutrition Threats 109

Chapter 13: Tactics to Avoid Nutrition Threats and Hit
Targets... 115

Conclusion: We're All Gonna Die 137

PART 1

MINDSET

Chapter 1

Your Brain Has Its Own Agenda

When you're in the business of death there is more on the line. Excuses, white lies, and saving face are not important. Regardless of rank or experience, a fighter pilot's only goal is to ensure the good guys stay alive and the bad guys don't. I've been flying fighters for over 12 years and all the fighter squadrons I've been in were filled with brilliant people dedicated to this one idea. The purpose of this book is to teach you to apply a fighter pilot mentality to your personal fitness. The same mindset and techniques that allow fighter pilots to perform consistently in high stress situations will help you to get and stay in the best shape of your life.

Several of my fellow pilots were killed in combat or unfortunate accidents. All fighter pilots have friends that were killed. This fact is integral to how we operate. I bet it's the same in other fighting forces. We can't accept mediocrity in ourselves or our squadron mates. The safety of men and women on the ground is also a concern. There have been many tragic fratricide accidents. Apart from dying, the scariest thing about combat is the thought that I could mess up and kill a good guy on the ground.

The resulting culture is very serious and sometimes immature. It's the stress. Pilots have a small margin for error and the missions require consistent performance. We train our new pilots like apprentices. We haze them and constantly watch and assess them. It's horrible to go through and I'm happy every day that I'm on the other side of the training table now. But I was taught the techniques and mindset necessary to pass the tests and move up the ranks. I also learned more techniques on my own. I didn't move up in a straight line. Sometimes I went sideways or even down, but I still made it to today. Now I train new F-16 fighter pilots as an old—at only 37—experienced pilot. I enjoy teaching the young students to be fighter pilots, but this book is not about how to be a fighter pilot. And it's not about how cool it is to be a fighter pilot. It's about applying some of the discipline and techniques I learned as a pilot, and now teach, to getting your body into the best shape it's ever been in.

I had always been in "okay" shape. Not great, not bad, just okay. I was not a college athlete, but in high school I played soccer at a high level and was a decent tennis player. I worked out in stretches of six months and would get in good shape. Amazingly, I ran an 8:45 mile and a half at the Academy when we had to run to class every day. But after that I just couldn't maintain a program. I couldn't stick to a healthy diet. I would always lose motivation and go back to eating bad food after a 12-hour flying day or drinking way too much beer in the fighter bar.

It wasn't until I started applying fighter pilot techniques to my own program that things started to change. I started setting targets and hitting them. I started tracking my workouts and I got what I was eating under control. I started teaching others the same techniques. When my good buddy said, "you changed my life," it was a turning point for me and the reason I wrote this book.

It's not rocket science

Every fighter pilot knows the KISS acronym. Keep It Simple Stupid. It's beaten into us from day one. Complicated plans are dangerous. The best plan is the simplest plan. Under combat stress and fatigue, even the best trained people make mistakes. The easier the plan is, the higher the chance of success.

Fighter pilot tactics are simple to remember and use. We remove the unnecessary parts of the problem and focus on a simple solution. This mentality is central to everything we do and is at the heart of this book. If ever in doubt, keep it simple stupid!

The techniques I outline in this book will follow this formula. They can be applied to any person at any age and in any physical or economic condition. They maximize the chance for success and minimize the chance for failure. I guarantee that these techniques will work for you if you put in the effort to follow them.

What's more valuable, the fighter jet or the pilot?

Is there anything you own more valuable than your body? I argue it is our most valuable asset. Which would you choose: everything you own burns to the ground or you die 10 years earlier?

If you chose option 2, you either have a really nice house or you don't value your life much. Yet we don't treat our bodies like our most valuable asset. I have friends who treat their cars like their life blood and their actual life blood like trash.

Compared to my body, my possessions are worthless. If my car breaks down I can ride a bus. If my house is destroyed, I can live with family or friends. But if my body breaks down, it's game over. I treat my body like a multi-million dollar fighter jet because, to me and my family, that's what it is, my most valuable tool.

A fighter jet is useless without a pilot, but if there is no jet around I can still fight. In a day you can train me to use a machine gun relatively effectively. You can't train a combat pilot in less than two years. They will just crash into the ground.

Getting in better shape is the best thing you can do to improve your most valuable asset. There are countless studies that definitively prove exercise and healthy eating increases the *quality* and *length* of your life. You will live *better* and *longer* with a healthy body. Getting in better shape is a war worth fighting. I will show you how to win that war step by step. But first you have to stop accepting excuses from the wimpy part of your brain.

These aren't the droids you're looking for...

At least three hours before each mission—in a small briefing room behind a locked security vault—the flight leader for the mission writes "Survive and Kill" on a large white briefing board. Under this main objective, in big blue marker he writes the mission-specific objectives that will make that possible. The goals go from big to small. "No good guy losses, all weapons released correctly, wingman stay with flight leads, correct communication" Whether it is 1v1 dogfighting or a 12v8 large force exercise, the flight lead stands in front of the objectives for an hour and explains on a whiteboard how the pilots will work together to survive and kill.

The pilots then fly the mission as close to the briefing as possible. Everything is filmed. After the flight they all watch the replay together. The flight lead watches critical phases in slow motion and assesses if the objectives are accomplished. If any objective isn't met—and there is usually at least one—they sometimes spend hours investigating why. After finding the cause, they decide on a solution. Younger pilots take notes and refer to the lessons later. This is how we constantly improve.

Now imagine you are a fighter pilot. Every day for 10 years, you spend hours planning, flying, and debriefing with one goal in mind, "Survive and Kill." How hard would it be for you to kill someone in combat? Would you hesitate to drop a bomb? I don't think you would because you are no different from us. We are normal men and women in an abnormal profession. I meet people all the time that tell me, "I couldn't be a fighter pilot and do what you do." But I believe without a doubt they could. I think anyone could, because it's all about consistent pressure over time.

You may be the nicest person in the world, but if you do something long enough and think something long enough your brain will change. I knew it was happening to me when I had nightmares in training. Enough time passed and the nightmares stopped. After that there were no second thoughts.

You can't trust your brain

If you think you're getting all the information, think again. Hold the book at arm's length and cover your right eye. Now stare at the X with your left eye and move the book closer to your face until the ● disappears.

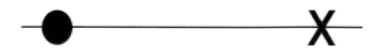

Now cover your left eye and stare at the ●. At the same distance from the image the X will disappear. We all have these two holes in our vision. They are caused by the biological cables (nerves) that run from the light-detecting cells in your retina to the processing section of your brain. Where the cable connects to your eye is the blind spot. You have lived your entire life with these two blind spots and chances are you didn't know it. We don't see a complete picture because our brain smooths out the image.

If an arrow was flying at your left eye from the ● and your right eye was closed you would never see the arrow. The image isn't smooth. Your brain is lying to you. It lies ALL THE TIME. It has its own agenda and often that agenda is neither healthy nor good for you. Since pilots started flying aircraft, we have been crashing into the ground because our brains thought the aircraft was doing one thing while it was actually doing something else. As instructors, we train students to never trust their biological sensors.

Which way is right?

After three winters in the Arctic cold of central Alaska my timing was lucky when an exchange assignment to Turkey showed up on the list. It was my time to move. I talked with my wife and we immediately chose Turkey. I was the only volunteer.

A year later I was in California at a military language school learning Turkish. My family and I then packed up for the seventh time in 12 years and made our way to Ankara. There I checked in with a Turkish F-16 squadron to fly as an instructor.

After a year in Turkey I was the instructor flying in the back seat of a young but capable Turkish wingman's jet. The student flies in the front seat and the instructor sits in the back seat. Once in a while I have to take the controls to show the proper way to do a maneuver or stop the student from flying into another plane. Otherwise the student flies and we watch. We call it riding trunk monkey. This flight was at night and it was his first flight using night vision goggles (NVGs). There was a grey cloud deck covering the base but the airspace we were going to was clear. The flight lead took off and 20 seconds later we followed him into the clouds. We attached the NVGs to our helmets, and the front pilot, Macit, started closing on the lead aircraft to "rejoin" with him and fly 10' formation off the lead's left wingtip.

As we flew closer to the lead jet, the lights of our aircraft illuminated the surrounding clouds in bright green flashes. Just as you may have seen in the movies, everything is green through NVGs. The flashes were bright and disorienting. Since we couldn't see the horizon or the ground, I knew without a doubt we were going to get spatially disoriented. I had been in similar situations before while crossing the ocean at night on a tanker. That night in Turkey, my brain was convinced we were turning, but since I wasn't flying I was able to look down and check the instruments. As I suspected, we were flying straight and level. I was disoriented and Macit confirmed my suspicions when he started flying too high on the lead aircraft. "Hocam, spatial disorienteyim," or *Teacher, I'm spatially disoriented.*

As instructors, we let the disorientation continue because it is important that the student experience his brain lying to him in a training environment. "Sakin ol," I said, *remain calm*. I told him to focus on his formation references: line up the wingtip missile with the intake, watch the spacing, and fly smooth. I helped him on the controls a little and we got back into the correct formation. A few minutes later we flew out of the clouds into clear air. Upon seeing the horizon, our brains reconfigured and we started to feel normal again.

Am I a better pilot than Macit? Absolutely not. He is an excellent pilot. I am just more experienced and have learned from my previous instructors not to trust my brain. Once you internalize that your brain often is wrong, it is much easier to do what is required. Macit will be better prepared when he gets spatially disoriented in the future.

Trusting your brain over your instruments is called "flying by the seat of your pants" and it will kill you. This is why so many non-professional pilots crash their private aircraft. Even highly trained professional pilots die due to spatial disorientation. When you get spatially disoriented it is hard as hell to trust what the instruments are saying. The reason is the "giant hand phenomenon." It happened to my buddy, who said "it felt as if a giant hand was holding my right arm on the controls." He used his left hand to grab the stick and recover the aircraft from the dive. How crazy is that? The rational trained part of his brain knew the aircraft was pointed at the ground in a death spiral but the irrational part of his brain stopped his arm from saving him. Using the other hand broke the spell.

Our brains don't give us all the details. Your brain will say "You can't see that arrow? No worries, it's not important." It also says things like "you don't need to get in shape, you're doing fine," or "one more beer's not gonna do any harm," or "go ahead, even though you are completely full, eat another dessert, you deserve it!" I call this part of the brain the wimpy voice because when it gets its way we act like giant wusses.

The wimpy voice is persuasive though, and knows you better than you know yourself. Most of the time, it doesn't even have to say anything because it is already part of your subconscious. It lives there, in your brain's blind spot. But once you know it's there you can learn to detect it and counteract it. Once you feel the spatial disorientation you are better prepared for it in the future.

The wimpy voice is not you. It is an artifact of your subconscious and will get in the way of reaching your goals. If you are spatially disoriented and don't recover the jet you will crash. Your brain knows this fact and still the wimpy voice can freeze your actions. It confuses and disorients. This book is a roadmap to overcoming the wimpy voice.

Are you ready for a little test? The program in this book takes 4 hours a week and the diet (or "food plan") is completely livable. Make a promise right now that you will do the complete program in this book.

Did you do it? Did you promise? I bet your first thoughts were some sort of excuse for why you can't do the program. Am I right? Take a second to think back. The first couple of thoughts were probably negative thoughts like "I don't have enough time, the author doesn't know what he's talking about, I'll probably get injured, it's too late for me..." This is the wimpy voice. The promise is not important. People promise stuff all the time. Then they don't do what they promised and feel bad about it and quit. Who are you promising anyway? The wimpy voice?

Break down and rebuild

You can be conditioned. It may take a long time, years even, but we can all be molded somewhat. Companies spend hundreds of billions of dollars on advertising because it works. In the military, indoctrination is part and parcel of our basic training, which doesn't actually involve the jobs new recruits will do in the military. The trainers even tell us the purpose of basic training is to break us down so they can rebuild us.

Everyone is susceptible to advertising, propaganda, indoctrination or whatever you want to call it. Our brains, like our bodies, can be molded. Why not use this fact to your advantage? Instead of letting other people manipulate you, why not convince yourself to achieve positive goals? All you have to do is focus on the task over a long enough time frame. In order to lead a rich and happy life, you must first learn to understand and control your own brain. You can do this through the medium of fitness.

"How can I persuade myself to get in shape?" How does anyone indoctrinate themselves? They tell themselves it is true every day. If 19 middle-aged idiots can brainwash themselves into flying fully loaded passenger planes into buildings, ultimately murdering kids and old people, I promise you can convince yourself that getting in shape is a priority.

It's not about making a promise to yourself. You don't promise that you'll brush your teeth; you just go and brush your teeth. The assumption is that you will brush your teeth. You don't have to convince anyone or make any compromises when it comes to brushing your teeth.

But how many years have you been compromising on getting in shape? How many years have you been on autopilot, unwilling to face the fact that a healthy life is a better life? How many years have you been eating and drinking whatever you want? You've eaten that food and drunk that drink a thousand times. Do you really need to eat it and drink it again? How many times have you said, "I need to get in shape?" How many times have you been drunk? How many times have you watched worthless TV shows and read crappy books? How many times have you been lazy and just lay on the couch watching other people make a positive impact on the world?

Now how many times have you been in impeccable shape, "ripped," even? How many times have you felt great and been amazed at what your body can accomplish? How many times have you set a difficult goal and tracked it to completion? How many times have you felt the confidence and motivation that seeing that goal to the end brings?

Chapter 2

Star Wars Is Better than *Top Gun*

Maybe it's generational but as far as I'm concerned, forget *Top Gun*, I'm a fighter pilot because of the original *Star Wars* trilogy (and maybe a little, *Last Starfighter*). In the final battle of the original *Star Wars* the rebels' task was to destroy the Death Star. If they accomplish this objective they win the battle. All friendly action was committed to this goal. Decoy the fighters, two torpedoes on the primary target and the Death Star explodes. During the bombing run, even as Darth Vader rolls in on his six and starts shooting his wingmen, Gold 5 pilot is saying "Stay on target." You must teach your brain to be completely focused on the task like the rebel fighters were focused on their bombing run.

Never mind the rebel fighters have poor defensive tactics and are just sitting ducks…at least they stayed on the target run. Imagine if Luke had broken off the attack and did not "stay on target." The rebels would have lost the battle and probably the war too. If you don't stay on target and develop a serious plan to reach one singular objective, your chance for success goes way down.

As a kid I was scared to death of the Terminator. Why was he so scary, besides having an indestructible skeleton and red eyes? Because, as John Conner yells, "He won't stop until you're dead. That's what he does…that's all he does!" What you program into the Terminator part of your brain is the task. Walls and police and fat friends may get in the way, but you don't care. It's what you do…it's all you do. Make the task a priority like the Terminator and stay on target even if Darth Vader rolls in on your six. If you stay focused on the task, have an open mind, and think in the long term, you literally cannot fail. Undoubtedly, there will be setbacks, but in the war to get in shape, in the long run, the only way you can fail is if you give up.

The information you are using is wrong

If you spend countless hours doing boring cardio and wonder why you "just can't lose weight," it is because our current model of eating calories and burning them is out to lunch. You don't burn calories. Your body is not a combustion engine.

Muscles don't burn anything. They contract by *breaking down* the chemical compound adenosine triphosphate (ATP). Your body gets ATP by *absorbing* food and converting it to glucose in the blood stream. Some of this glucose is converted to ATP and sent to the muscle cells. The rest of the glucose is stored in the muscles as glycogen (sugar), in the blood as blood sugar, and as fat in your midsection.

When you command your muscles to contract, a cell has three options. It can use the limited amount of ATP it has directly, it can use the limited amount of glycogen it has by turning it into ATP, or it can activate the aerobic system and get sustained long-term energy. The first two processes are ancient, inefficient, and anaerobic, which means they don't need oxygen. Bacteria use these processes. We, however, have evolved to use the two ancient processes *and* a third aerobic process.

The reason you don't lose weight is because the aerobic process is 15 times more efficient than the anaerobic processes. The aerobic process makes 37 ATP molecules while the anaerobic processes make only 2 ATP molecules *from the same glucose molecule.* This is why high-intensity interval training (HIIT) cardio is more effective than regular cardio, because it forces the body to use anaerobic processes.

It gets worse. The Atwater system we currently use to find calories—4 calories per gram of carbohydrates and protein and 9 calories per gram of fat—was developed in the 1890s. While Wilbur Wright was test-flying the Wright Flyer, Wilbur Atwater was burning food in a box and measuring the heat as calories. We aren't flying in airplanes made out of paper, sticks, and bicycle gears. Why are we still putting our food in a box and lighting it on fire? No wonder there is an obesity epidemic.

If the basic assumptions are wrong, how have so many thousands of people gotten in amazing shape? What do the models on fitness magazines do that you don't do? They found a system that worked for them. I want to teach you how you can find a system that works for you using tried and true fighter pilot techniques.

The 4Ts

I learned the 4Ts during my best experience so far in the military, on a training exercise called the Tactical Leadership Programme. I went to this month-long exercise in 2006 when it was located in a small rural town in Belgium, on an air base nestled in a forest surrounded by green countryside and French-speaking villages.

Over the next 4 weeks another U.S. pilot and I flew all over Europe with British, German, Italian, French, Spanish, and Czech pilots. After simulating bombing runs against a German frigate over the North Sea we returned to Belgium and drank Belgian beer while laughing with the Germans and Italians in the bar; the next day we flew to France against other air and land targets and drank French wine and ate French cheese; the day after was Spain and eating paella.

I will never forget the foreign pilots I flew with. One German Tornado pilot had been an East German military policeman before the wall fell: "It was great fun." He sounded exactly like Arnold Schwarzenegger and had the same square jaw, "we would walk around and find a riot or something and beat some people, then we would train on machine guns and later go to the bars…it was great."

My favorite quote from an Italian pilot (and there were many) was: "Italians never beg for sex…we take it or we pay for it." He then immediately broke into a heartfelt rendition of "With or Without You" by U2. I heard every painful note of it clearly, because we had packed four of us into the back of a small European rental car.

The exercise was during the World Cup. This only increased the magnitude of the event as I watched firsthand each country's reaction to the losses and victories. The Italian pilots didn't say a word after their country won the cup, but somehow their proud arrogance bled through. The fact they were wearing the Italian National Team Jersey *over* their flight suits may also have helped.

The technique that the practiced European instructors taught us—and which never let me down in exercises later in Alaska and Turkey—was the 4Ts. Each morning we showed up to the mass briefing room at 8:00 and the instructors told us which country we were flying to. Somehow, 4 hours later, 26 aircraft from seven different countries took off and flew a large force coordinated mission. How do you make a tactical plan that quickly with so many countries involved? How do you ensure 100% safety for all parties? We did exactly what the instructors told us to do and we slammed the Red forces.

- **Task**: Primary objective of the entire mission. Examples are "Defend Blueland from air aggression," "Degrade enemy command and control," "Destroy enemy combat capability."
- **Targets**: Based on intel, if we hit these targets we will accomplish the task.
- **Threats**: Based on intel, these are the threats that can stop us from hitting the targets.
- **Tactics**: The specific techniques that we will use to avoid the threats and hit the targets.

The blueprint of this book is the 4Ts. This technique enables me to efficiently explain the objective, identify what can get in the way, and describe the best plan of attack for you to get and stay in the best shape of your life.

I flew in several exercises where the mission commander (MC) chose the tactics himself and micromanaged the planning process. He did not double tap (bomb by separate assets) the primary targets, the surface-to-air missiles (SAMs) were not suppressed, and the air cover assets did not focus their air defense in the right area. We lost several good guys (simulated), missed important targets, and had long, painful debriefs.

On the flip side, I witnessed excellent mission commanders who used the 4Ts. These MCs used all the resources of the group by asking pointed questions. They knew they didn't know everything and allowed other people to contribute to the plan. Everyone knew the primary task. The group selected the most effective targets and all the threats were identified. If the task, targets, and threats are correctly identified, developing the tactics isn't that difficult. It is laying the groundwork and correctly following the 4Ts that builds an effective game plan.

Make sure your mind is open to other ways to accomplish the task. Although the MC has the final say, good commanders listen to inputs and then decide the best course of action. There is more than one way to destroy a target. Do we even have to destroy it? Can we go around it to achieve our objective? As long as we have a clearly defined task then we know where to end up.

I have never seen an exercise or combat mission go exactly according to plan. We've gotten close, but there is always something: thunderstorms, radio malfunctions, surprise enemy actions, incorrect intelligence, or plain old human error. The successful people in life have learned to avoid these roadblocks (threats) to consistently achieve their short-range goals (targets). As long as these goals are chosen correctly, they will reach the long-term objective (task). All successful people use some form of this process whether they know it or not. I will show you in this book how to use the combat-proven 4Ts in your own life to stay on target and get the body you've always wanted.

The OODA loop

In any fighter squadron you will hear jokes about the OODA (pronounced "oo-da") loop. Specifically you will hear "get inside their OODA loop." The OODA loop is unique among military acronyms, because it is not a TLA (three letter acronym). If this theory were created today, I think its developer, Colonel John Boyd, would have chosen ODA loop instead. Like all other military acronyms, the OODA loop has to have a sexy acronym so we can use it in clever sentences like "my kid got inside my OODA loop." This means "my kid was able to think faster and out-analyze me, once this happens she can foresee my actions and there is nothing I can do to win."

OODA stands for Observe, Orient, Decide, and Act. In the OODA loop, we objectively *observe* what is happening, *orient* ourselves by looking at the options, *decide* on an option, and then *act* on it. We keep repeating this process in a loop. After we act, we observe the results, orient, decide, and act again. If we do this loop faster and more accurately than our adversary, we "get inside their OODA loop." The most important part of the OODA loop and why I am explaining it to you is: *you must objectively track your progress.*

You have to write useful, accurately measured information down in a log. If you don't objectively and accurately observe your progress you can't start a decision loop process. You will stop productive techniques that are moving you closer to your goal and instead start unproductive techniques. From my experience this is the main reason people quit, they don't track their progress. If you are not willing to track your workouts by writing them down or if you can't track your weight and waist size weekly, then I recommend you don't waste your time starting.

In Turkey I trained a young Turkish sergeant named Yigit. After working out in the gym for a few months on his own and not seeing much progress he asked me to help him. After three weeks of starting my program he approached me and said he was losing his motivation. A friend of Yigit's had joked with him: "You work out all the time? You look fatter!"

"Let's take a look at your notebook," I said. His goal was to lose fat. According to his logbook, in the past week he had lost half an inch from his waist, but his weight had gone up a pound. I could also tell from the log that his strength had increased. He had lifted more weight than the week before. This told me immediately that not only was he losing fat, he was also gaining muscle at the same time. He was making great progress and was on target to reach his goal within a month. After we looked at the numbers together, he continued the program and achieved his goal.

Coincidentally, the following week I had the same feeling that Yigit had. While trying to lose fat, I too thought my progress had stopped. I didn't feel any skinnier, but when I looked back in my logbook I was surprised—just like the Turkish sergeant—to see that I was still on my progress line. I was hitting the targets. Like recovering from spatial disorientation, I had to convince my brain to look at the numbers and see the truth. If I hadn't tracked my progress I probably would have changed a program that was already effective.

Chapter 3

True Change is Long-Term

The Air Force does not take a kid right out of college and put him in a combat fighter aircraft. There is a step by step process. Candidates first start out in Cessna aircraft for a private pilot's license. Then come jet propeller aircraft, fighter jet trainers, and finally, combat fighters. It takes an intense steady progression over more than two years to create a fighter pilot. And then they are still just dangerous enough to be the F'ing New Guy (FNG) in a fighter squadron. It takes another 2 years before they are experienced enough to lead other wingmen around.

It would be crazy to put someone directly into a multi-million dollar fighter and expect them to fly it safely, much less fight with it. We will apply the same mentality with your body. Every day your body will get a teeny-tiny bit stronger. You will lose a small amount of fat. Your cardiovascular system will become stronger by a small percentage. Your joints, ligaments, and connective tissue will be just a tad more resilient. The ATP, creatine, and glycogen in your muscles will recover a microscopic bit faster. But as the days and weeks pass, and then the months, the canyon will start to form and the water will start to run faster down the river. As the water flows faster, the gains will come a little quicker. You will be able to work harder. You will gain a deeper understanding of your body and what diet it needs for maximum performance. You will have developed systems and habits that counteract the negative habits of the past. After a year you will have completely changed your mindset and your body.

A year! How can it possibly take that long? Well...it depends on your goals, it could take less or more time, but it will take time. This is why people fail. They think too short term, their goals are too small. You need to have ambition and self confidence in what you can accomplish. This is why getting started is the first task. You must commit to a plan and then follow through to achieve the goal. This process will reinforce itself in your brain. The more you follow the plan, the more results you will see. The more results you see, the more you will follow the plan. Getting in shape is the most attainable task. The only thing between the current you and a slim, strong body, is you. No matter what anyone says, you control what food goes in your mouth and what activities you do.

Consistent pressure is unstoppable

In my 13-year career as a fighter pilot, 85% of the pilots I have worked with are average fighter pilots and 15% are exceptional. Among such dedicated and trained individuals I consider being average a compliment. I hope I am considered average by my peers.

This means that out of the 100 or so pilots I have worked closely with on a daily basis I consider 15 of them exceptional. Out of these 15, I believe only one pilot was naturally an amazing pilot. He was just better at everything. Maybe he worked harder when I wasn't looking but he appeared to simply be better than the rest of us. When we went go-cart racing, he always won. When we went skiing, he was the best. He won every game of twister. He is also ridiculously nice and wears a cheery Christmas sweater with a fuzzy reindeer on it during the holiday season. My point is that the other 14 were not naturally better pilots. They just consistently worked harder than everyone else.

I grew up playing video games. Against my parents' wishes I would bike 2 miles down to the local Dairy Queen. With two quarters I found in the couch I could easily play for 30 minutes.

This dedication to video games served me well in pilot training. I won "best hands" in fighter training and won all air-to-air and air-to-ground events. I finished number 1 out of 11 pilots. The problem is that sometimes success limits us. It made me cocky and I performed below my potential on my first few assignments.

The truly exceptional pilots trained harder and longer than I did in the 12 years after pilot training. While I was drinking in the bar, they were training in the simulator. When I went home early on Friday night (7 PM), they stayed to hear combat stories from the senior pilots. When I watched TV on Sunday, they went into work. They simply made being a great fighter pilot more of a priority. They wanted it more, so each day they spent a little more time than I did training, studying, and thinking about it. I still put in at least 60-hour weeks training and studying, but they spent a little more time than all of us each day and in the end became truly exceptional combat pilots.

I watched consistent pressure over time change a below-average pilot into an exceptional pilot. The Top Gun pilot in one of my squadrons had finished last in his training class, but it just made him work harder after pilot training. You don't have to give up weekends or time with your family to get in shape, but you do have to give consistent priority to the task.

For instance, there will be times when a friend will offer you your favorite junk food while you are trying to lose weight. If you can't resist, then I say go ahead and eat it, but don't go to the store and buy a box of it to keep at your house. You can always take a short break or fit cheat days into your food plan. In fact, we will plan break weeks and cheat days into your program.

I listen to my body and take a week off when required. It happens every two to three months. I'm taking a break week right now. My joints and muscles are recovering, but the best part is that next week I will be excited to get back into my workout.

Also, one day a week of bad eating is not going to affect your overall food plan.[1] If you maintain a healthy diet 85% (6/7days)

---

[1] See Brandon Carter, *Ultimate Cuts:7 Secrets to Burn Fat Fast as Hell* (Amazon Digital, 2014). Also check out Carter's many videos at www.youtube.com/user/HighLifeWorkout. He is

of the time, I promise you will reach your goals. But you have to eat healthy 85% of the time *consistently*. Maybe you were in amazing shape in high school or college, but I guarantee there are tens of thousands of people your age who are in better shape. Why? Because they have made getting a well-muscled, healthy body a priority over a longer period of time.

It's not you that wants to quit. It's the wimpy part of your brain. Just tell yourself this is the task. The task is the priority. Every day dedicated to the task chips a little more stone from the canyon. Cheat and modify if you have to, but don't quit. As an example, take a look at a log scale for the Dow Jones stock market over the last 100 years.

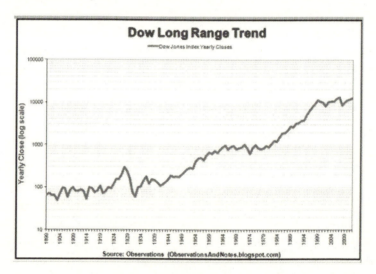

Observations Blog (www.observationsandnotes.blogspot.com)

If you zoom in on the monthly returns, you see extreme ups and downs. Even in the yearly chart there is a lot of variation. But imagine if the stock market "quit" after the Great Depression of 1929. The stock market would have missed the greatest creation of wealth in the history of the world. You will undoubtedly have

---

very convincing about the value of compound movements and the importance of a cheat day. I learned about the cave man portion method, discussed in Chapter 13, from Carter's work. His workout blog can be viewed here: http://www.brandoncarter.com.

variation in your own program. Sometimes you will go backwards. That's okay, just don't quit. Think about the exceptional combat pilots, the stock market, and the Grand Canyon.

If you focus on this single goal your body has no choice but to adapt. The pressure that you need to apply is not as great as you think. The pivotal factor is that you stay on target and maintain a slight upward trajectory in the long term.

Find your inner vanity

There is a motto in the fighter pilot community: "If you're not cheating, you're not trying." It means we will do anything to win *within the rules of the game*. Watch any professional athlete such as a football or basketball player. They grab their opponent's jersey at key times and stand in front of charging players in order to get knocked to the ground. They foul the opponent to avoid a score. Would they do these things if they weren't completely focused on the task? Use anything *within the rules of the game* to your advantage.

If the goal in your mind is to "get in better shape," I encourage you to think more like a fighter pilot. Make your goal more measurable, like "I want a 6-pack" or "I want my body fat percentage to be 10% (17% for women)." Be ambitious with the goal and use vanity to your advantage. Everyone has an ego and is self-conscious. You care about your appearance and what other people think about you. It's impossible not to. Women put on makeup and men shave every day. There is a reason that every fitness magazine has at least one article on losing belly fat. We care about our appearance and most people care about having a flat stomach. The desire to have a great looking body is a motivational lever we can press to reach a positive goal: a healthy mind and body.

Now don't overdo it. This may come as a surprise, but more than a few fighter pilots I know have been considered arrogant. I certainly was after fighter training. Success went to my brain and limited me. There is a big difference between arrogance and having a positive self-image. Arrogance doesn't let us listen to other points of view. We can always be wrong. Only the arrogant can't acknowledge their shortcomings.

My back hurts...I must be getting old

Nope, you're just weak. Now I am not a doctor, I am a fighter pilot, so if you have any genuine medical concerns please see a medical professional. That being said, from my experience doctors are clueless when it comes to joint health, shoulder issues, and especially back pain. In fact the North American Spine Society even admits they don't know what is going on: "Many different theories try to explain chronic [low back] pain. The exact mechanism is not completely understood." [2] In their defense, they do recommend weight loss, stretching, and strength training as the solution.

How many people do you know who suffer from lower back pain? I know a lot. In fact, half of *all* working Americans admit to having experienced back pain symptoms in the past year. Are you kidding me? That means there is a 50% chance that you had lower back pain symptoms in the past year. Back pain is something I wouldn't wish on my enemy (well maybe) and undoubtedly lowers quality of life. Now imagine your life with less back pain. Imagine everything in the world weighs less. How much money or time would you give to get this?

Ever notice how movers can lift a ton of weight with no apparent ill effects to their backs? We move a lot in the military and I am always amazed at how strong these guys are. I have a desk that I swear weighs 200 lb. and the movers casually pick it up and load it on the truck. Ever notice how strong farmers and laborers are? How many of these people have chronic lower back pain? Half? I doubt it.

According to a scholarly review of surveys about lower back pain conducted in the mid- to late-twentieth century, high-

---

[2] "Chronic Low Back Pain," North American Spine Society Public Education Series (2009): http://www.knowyourback.org/Documents/chronic_lbp.pdf

income countries have much higher rates of back pain than lower and middle income countries:

> Specifically, rates are 2-4 times higher among Swedish, German, and [Belgian] general populations than among Nigerian, southern Chinese, Indonesian, and Filipino farmers. Within low-income countries, rates [of back pain] are higher among urban populations than among rural populations...[3]

If our medical technology is so much more advanced, why do we have twice the incidence of lower back pain? You may argue that there are fewer doctors in Nigeria. Maybe they have the same amount of back pain, but they just don't complain? The rebuttal is that in Nigeria, farmers have reported less back pain than the city dwellers. This tells me that the rural laborers simply have stronger backs.

If your back is strong from doing manual labor (or working out) you will be less likely to hurt it in your other daily activities. If your back is weak from sitting at a desk all day at work and then watching TV all night consistently, when you *do* have to lift something your weak back muscles and ligaments will let your spine down and cause an injury.

My mom broke her back in a car accident. The first exercise every doctor gives her is a stomach crunch or a reverse back extension. It never works. In weight lifting we don't curve our backs. Watch an Olympic deadlifter or squatter on YouTube. How many of them have curved backs during their lifts? The current world record deadlift is 1015 lb.! These athletes lift three times their body weight off the ground, yet when we pick up 50 lb. we're worried about hurting our backs.

Practice good form

What is the difference between us and Olympic deadlifters? For one, form. They always keep their back straight when lifting

---

[3] Ernest Violinn, "The Epidemiology of Low Back Pain in the Rest of the World: A Review of Surveys in Low- and Middle-Income Countries," *Spine* 22, no. 15 (1997): 1747; 1752.

a lot of weight. Their muscles are also tightened and they have their diaphragm full. This forms a natural weight belt around the lower back. The second difference is strength. Their muscles and connective tissues are simply stronger than yours and mine.

We can improve form and strength, like everything else in life, with practice. Resistance training—no matter your age or sex—will improve your life because it will make your back stronger. For this reason alone, I believe getting in shape is important. Devote one month to your program and note the changes in your life. Continue for six months and you will be amazed at the difference in your daily life. Make it a habit and it will change your life. I know it has changed mine.

Fighter pilots pull a lot of gravitational forces, or G's as we call them. When anything changes direction it accelerates. When you go around a turn in a car you are pulling lateral Gs. You are accelerating sideways into the door. When you feel heavy at the bottom of a roller coaster you are pulling maybe 2 G's. Fighter aircraft are designed to pull up to nine times the ordinary force of gravity because this is basically the maximum force a human can endure. At 9 G forces you weigh nine times your 1 G weight standing on Earth. A 200 lb. man weighs 1800 lb. at 9 Gs, and a 100 lb. woman weighs 900 lb. When we do high-G flights such as dogfighting, the capillaries in our forearms break. We cleverly call them geasles since they look like measles bumps but are caused by high G forces.

The most G's I ever pulled was in a base competition called a Turkey Shoot. I was flying as an Aggressor in Alaska. In the competition we were flying as the Red-Air, or simulated enemy, for another base that had F-15s and F-22s. As Red-Air we weren't necessarily in the competition, but we are fighter pilots and a competition is a competition. We wanted to win our fights. We had no external tanks or anything else on the jet. Imagine a stripped-down race car. The jet was light and still had the same amount of thrust from a large inlet GE-made engine. Also, the ice cold Arctic air is very dense, which allows the engine to pull in more air to create more thrust. Combine all these things and it's like riding a bull at the rodeo. Hang on and squeeze your legs as hard as you can in an anti-G straining maneuver to not pass out. If you don't maintain blood pressure to your brain by holding your breath and squeezing your large leg muscles, you will go unconscious for up to 30 seconds. Since we are flying at a speed of 10 miles a minute, it is better to be conscious.

The setup was 1v1 dogfighting starting from a head-on pass. As Red-Air, we didn't know until the merge if we would be fighting a legacy F-15 or the brand new F-22. I talked to the other pilot on the radio prior to the merge. Based on his call sign, I assumed he was an F-15. I saw the jet 6 miles away as a small dot on the horizon. I was pumped up to win and lit the afterburner. I aimed my jet slightly right of the dot to pass within 1000' nose-to-nose, like a jousting match. At a mile every 3 seconds, he blew by me 18 seconds later at a combined 1000 mph. It was an F-22! I had finally gotten the chance to dogfight one.

I called "Fights on" to begin the engagement and rolled my jet across his tail and tried to pull the stick off. In that cold Arctic air, I G-strained against 9 Gs for over 18 seconds. I focused on squeezing my legs as hard as I could and on doing quick air exchanges every 3 seconds to keep blood going to my brain. In the air, all I remember thinking is that I had to win. The strategy is like 3-dimensional bumper cars. Turn around in a circle faster than the other guy. You can bump him from the side and he can't bump you.

If you are going 500 mph around the circle and pulling more Gs than the jet (or your body) should be able to handle, it doesn't matter what the other aircraft is, you are going to go around the circle faster. I pointed first and simulated a missile shot. But an F-22 in capable hands is a truly amazing machine. Even though I won the engagement, we continued fighting and he had no problem winning easily.

Although that was a lot of Gs it is a common occurrence. All pilots have stories about pulling high Gs. We are constantly under G while turning our heads and torsos to find the adversary or our wingmen. This puts a lot of strain on our necks and lower backs.

Several pilots I know fly with lower back support pillows; otherwise they get excruciating back pain. Once every couple of months a pilot will come in unable to turn his head. It's happened to me twice. I also had lower back pain on and off for 3 years.

Then I started doing exercises to strengthen my lower back, specifically deadlifts and squats. I have since had zero episodes in the jet. Once, while deadlifting, my back started to hurt so I stopped and took a few days off. I was fine three days later.

A good fighter pilot friend of mine had the same results. He is no longer scared to pick up heavy objects and has no problem pulling high Gs. Both my 66-year old mother and 67-year old father saw huge benefits in strength and pain relief by doing those exercises as well. Focus on the task and start slow. It will take a few months to strengthen your core muscles and connective tissues but once you get them in shape you will be amazed at what you can accomplish. Stop wasting time on less efficient ways to improve your life. Imagine you are confronting the threat head-on. Turn across its tail and pull for all you're worth. Let's get started with the program.

PART 2

WORKOUT

Chapter 4

Task 1: Start, Maintain, and Track a Training Program

How much willpower does it take to brush your teeth every night? I'm guessing zero. I bet you don't even think about brushing your teeth while you are brushing your teeth. You don't convince yourself to brush your teeth. You just walk in the bathroom and brush your teeth. When you forget to brush your teeth and realize it while you are already in bed, what do you do? I know what I do. I lay there for a few seconds disappointed in myself for forgetting something so mundane. Then for 10 seconds or so, I consider not brushing my teeth. Images of decaying teeth, dentists, and cavities come into my mind. I grudgingly get up and brush my teeth. Then I lie back down with a refreshed mouth and a sense of accomplishment.

On a normal day it takes me zero willpower to go to the gym. I don't plead with my wimpy voice. I just stand up and physically move my body into a workout location. Once in a while I don't want to go, but I still go. If I really can't make it to the gym one day then I make up for it another day. Am I different from you? Not at all, I used to struggle too. Why is it so nice to sleep in when we don't have to do something, like go to school or work? I believe our bodies have evolved to maximize energy efficiency.

Focus on consistency, not intensity

In *The New York Times* bestseller *Willpower: Rediscovering the Greatest Human Strength*, Roy F. Baumeister and John Tierney describe a psychological study of marathon runners which reveals some interesting insight into how willpower is relative to the task at hand. One group of runners was told at the start of the marathon that they would have to run one additional mile for a total of 27 miles. A second group of runners was told the same thing, but at the finish line. They thought they had finished a grueling race, only to then be given the bad news that they had to run yet another mile. The first group, which knew at the beginning, ran the 27-mile race faster than the second group who only learned at the end. Slower runners in the first group outran faster runners in the second group.

The study shows that we conserve willpower based on the length of the task. Weaker marathon runners were mentally prepared to go the longer distance and could force their bodies to endure. The stronger runners exhausted all their willpower and did not have enough mental or physical energy to continue at a reasonable pace. This is why so many workouts and crash diets fail. The brain musters a certain amount of willpower to achieve a task based on expectations of its length. When that time is up, as with 30-day cleanses or 30-day workouts, our willpower is depleted and, like the marathon runners, we quit. They didn't technically quit, but they ran a lot slower.

The purpose of this task is to make going to the gym four times a week the same as brushing your teeth. In the end you won't have to plead with your wimpy voice. You won't have to deplete your willpower. You will simply work out. For those times you don't or can't go, you will make yourself go or you will make it up the very next day. If you have to make the workout easier or shorter to make this happen, so be it.

Task 1: Start, Maintain, and Track a Training Program	
Primary targets:	1. Work out 4 days a week or more. 2. Write down sets, reps, and weight each workout; write down weekly weight and waist measurements.
Threats:	Lack of time, motivation, knowledge, money, too late to start.
Tactics:	Warm up 5 min, Stretch 5 min, Compound resistance training workout (25 min), Cardio (15 min. steady-state or 8 min. of HIIT). **Total=50 minutes or 43 minutes with HIIT**

In the fighter community, we call all the required items going to and from a fight "admin." It is basically fighter pilot paperwork. It is boring and takes energy but it has to be done well so we can get to the real training. Good pilots have solid admin. Every mission, we have to start, check in with each other on the radio, taxi, and take-off all timed to the second. We normally fly as 2 or 4 aircraft formations, so improper admin wastes training time and taxpayer money. Poor admin is an indication of fatigue, poor preparation, or task saturation. If we miss radio check-ins during a large exercise it can delay the entire 50-ship package. If a student pilot can't handle admin in a trainer aircraft they are washed out. The first six months of pilot training is all admin training. We hammer solid admin into the students, and you need to do the same. We want to put your workout admin on autopilot. We don't want willpower to be involved. If we can take willpower out of the equation then there is nothing to exhaust.

- **Step 1**: Overcome any mental blocks you may have to working out. It is just the wimpy voice. Ignore it.
- **Step 2**: Select a training routine that you will follow and get a small notebook and pen.
- **Step 3**: Choose one of the programs I recommend in this book or pick a different one, as long as it is trackable. You can always change programs later if you don't like the one you are doing. I change every 3-4 months.
- **Step 4:** Make sure you prepare your gym bag or have the clothes you need for working out at home. This is the start to good admin. Don't give your wimpy voice a chance to shout out a lame excuse.

While serving in Turkey a Turkish conscript named Mehmet asked if I could help him. All Turkish males have to serve in the military: 6 months if they went to college or 12 months if they didn't. He was serving 6 months. Mehmet had never worked out before and said he used to be overweight. He had lost the weight but didn't have any muscle.

"Teacher, can I get muscle?" he asked in a quiet voice.

"Of course," I said, "you already have it, we just have to make it stronger."

I wrote out a basic food plan and weight program that consisted of body weight squats, sit-ups, and push-ups. After a week I asked how the program was going. He said he didn't like it because the push-ups were too hard. I had him try a couple push-ups and realized that he didn't have the strength yet to do a full push-up.

I bent down next to him in the hallway. "You're not strong enough yet, start by doing push-ups from your knees."

"That's embarrassing…"

"Mehmet, all you have to do is keep up the knee push-ups for two or three weeks and then you can forever after do real push-ups."

He didn't seem to get it and quit the next week. He refused to do the knee push-ups. I tried talking him into going to the gym, but he "didn't have the time." If he had fought through just two weeks of embarrassment, he would have been able to do actual push-ups, for once in his life, and would have been well on his way to being in great shape.

Start at the beginning

If I see overweight or weak people in a gym, I am happy they are there. They are doing something to change their lives and I honestly hope they continue. But I know that a lot of them won't. The people that definitely won't continue are the ones sweating too much and breathing too hard. If you're not in shape you can undoubtedly get there, but it isn't going to happen in a week or even a month. You need to take your time. Arnold Schwarzenegger started at the beginning and so should you.

We all start at the beginning. Every single person in the world who has ever been in great shape at one point in life was a newbie, wandering aimlessly around the gym asking dumb questions and doing the exercises incorrectly. It is completely fine to ask questions. It is completely fine if you're not in shape and you fumble around with the exercises. The point of being in a gym, on a track, or in any other fitness venue is to improve your fitness.

Even if you have already been working out I still recommend the same program, but you can use shorter rest times and supersets of the upper body exercises. Supersets are two different exercises back-to-back without rest in between. For instance, one set of bench presses and then immediately do one set of lat pull-downs. I consider a workout program successful if it maximizes benefit in minimum workout time and is simple to track and execute. In the end it must be something that you will do on a continual basis.

I would have loved to see Mehmet in the gym knocking out push-ups and being proud with his goofy grin. He was a great guy but I just couldn't make him do it. He couldn't make himself do it. The wimpy part of his brain had taken control and ruined his plans. He'd really wanted it. He could have just done a different exercise, but he found an excuse instead.

Whenever I hear people like Mehmet say they want to be in better shape, or they want to lose weight, I immediately think "go and do it then." But there is always an excuse isn't there? I don't even hear excuses anymore. All I hear is, "I wanted to perform *but* excuse, excuse, excuse, *because* excuse, excuse, excuse." Only your mom cares about your excuses and deep down, she probably doesn't care either. Honestly, no one cares why you couldn't get something done. All that matters is the results, and if they are consistently bad, you are doing something wrong. It is not the rest of the world's fault.

This mentality is hammered home in a fighter squadron. Starting in basic training if the required result isn't achieved, our answer can only be, "No excuse, sir." If you couldn't make it happen then you didn't try hard enough. You didn't cheat enough. You didn't stack every advantage in your corner to make losing impossible. Even when the instructors made it impossible to accomplish the task, which was often, they still only allowed the response "No excuse, sir." It is a mentality we were forced to internalize and you should as well.

You must learn to be honest and never give yourself excuses. An excuse means you don't accept responsibility for the outcome, but blame outside forces instead. There will always be roadblocks, there will always be difficulties—but there will not be excuses. Just find the root cause of the problem, change the behavior, and move on. Find out why it didn't happen for you and fix it. If you didn't have clothes for the gym, put an extra set in your car. If you didn't have time to do your workout, then change it so it's shorter and you can do it at home. If your shoulder hurts, do a leg workout or run. There is always a way to win. Just like Luke Skywalker didn't give up in the trench of the Death Star, a fighter pilot never gives up. There is always a chance Han Solo will swoop in and blast Darth Vader's ship at the last second. Even in the worst position anything can happen. The enemy gun can jam, the missile can fail to fuse, or the radar can lose its lock on the target.

You don't have to be a fighter pilot to have perseverance and mental fortitude. Just imagine yourself never giving up. Then keep imagining yourself never giving up. Imagine yourself imagining yourself never giving up. How do you think I wrote this book? Fighter pilots are known for drinking and telling stories in the bar, not writing books. It was difficult, but I just told myself every day that I wouldn't give up. The key is to focus on the task and learn how your brain works. Learn how you can manipulate it. Your brain is not as unchangeable as you think.

Chocolate-covered deer poop

I starved in the woods during survival training for two weeks and my brain changed. I ate boiled rabbit heart, ants, and stole beef jerky from the instructors. I would not do any of those things under normal circumstances.

A week into the program, our two cadet instructors brought my group to a clearing in the woods. There they had set up a tepee with hundreds of beef jerky strips hanging from horizontal strings. While standing in front of rows of delicious-looking beef jerky, the non-starved instructors explained the process of making beef jerky while hiding from the enemy in the wilderness. I remember thinking how handy this information would be if I got shot down and needed to find a random meaty animal to turn into jerky. At the end of the presentation the instructors were kind enough to give us each a single piece of jerky.

When you are starving, it is better to not have any food than a single one-inch piece of delicious beef jerky. During the next station, I looked back and saw the rows of beef jerky unattended. I pointed this out to my buddy Jimmy next to me. Like we were taught, we escaped and evaded from the next station and low crawled to the tepee. It was like two foxes in a hen house. I filled my pockets with beef jerky and ate it silently on the trail back to camp. Unfortunately, when you are starving, even 20 pieces of one-inch beef jerky is just a drop in the bucket.

My friend Sharpie ate deer droppings. The instructors had secretly placed tactical Milk Duds around a pile of deer poop. They then "found" the poop while leading the students through the woods. The chance encounter gave them the opportunity to explain that deer droppings are edible. They both then ate the Milk Duds as proof, calmly saying "not bad really." Sharpie was from the farm country of Colorado and was hungry enough to try it. "Tastes like grass" he said, "a little stringy though." He was upset when he later found out about the Milk Duds.

You don't have to starve yourself to change your brain but you do have to apply consistent pressure over time. Think of the 18-milewide Grand Canyon. A few flash floods didn't carve out that gully. Everything is changeable with enough pressure over time.

In the Air Force, when we dig deeper into any task, we also ask ourselves if we are able to do it. Is the task achievable with our current forces? If the enemy has too many air assets then we may take heavy losses and end up losing the war. If we don't have enough suppression assets for the enemy surface-to-air missiles (SAMs) then the same may be true. If the task will win the war, then we may still proceed even if the risks are high.

For the first task of "Start, Maintain, and Track a Training Program," the answer to the question of whether we can do it is yes. No matter your age or current level of fitness, starting a training program can and should be done tomorrow.

The key to victory on this task is consistent pressure over time. It's not about killing yourself in the gym for a few weeks. You will quit. I would quit. Your habits will change, but they won't change in one day or a week. With consistent pressure we will coax fat off one cell at a time and build muscle one cell at a time. We won't try to do both at the same time. If in doubt, remember to keep it simple, stupid, and focus on the task. If you have to choose between an activity that moves you towards the task or doing something else, choose the activity that gets you closer to your goal. To complete the task all you have to do is hit the targets.

Chapter 5

Workout Targets

The United Arab Emirates pilot turned away from the mission commander whiteboard and said to the 28 of us in the briefing, "That is the strike plan, any questions?" I couldn't hold my tongue and raised my hand and asked, "Can Gazelle flight bomb the SA-2? We fly near it on the way to our targets." In the playback on PowerPoint our 4-ship of F-16s flew right by the surface-to-air missile (SAM). "Why not use two of our eight bombs and hit the SAM? All our targets are inside its threat ring."

The MC was annoyed. This was the second time I had brought up this idea and he hadn't approved it the first time. It wasn't even my idea, my Turkish wingman had thought of it. The SAM wasn't that capable, but it was right in the middle of the damn scenario. It was like the shield on the Death Star.

"The SA-2 is already being targeted by the F-4s," he said in a flat tone. "The other F-16 flight will shoot anti-radiation missiles at the SAM and the F-4s will destroy it with long-range missiles. Are there any other questions?" He looked around the room, which was quiet now.

During the mission two of the four F-4s targeting the SAM had an emergency and returned to base. The other two were shot down by an enemy fighter before they launched their missiles (all simulated of course). The SAM remained operational and slaughtered our train of strike aircraft one-by-one as we entered the threat ring.

That SAM was a primary target but we didn't treat it like one. The MC decided to prioritize secondary targets over double-targeting the SAM. With that SAM operational, like the Death Star force shield, we can't achieve our mission.

You must choose the right targets. If hitting the targets doesn't allow us to accomplish the task then we have chosen incorrectly. The first primary target is four days of workouts a week. I've found that four days a week is enough to see real progress, but not too much that it takes over your life. Until you, your friends and family, and your boss and coworkers realize that working out is just a part of what you do, it will be hard to make time to work out. You not only have to train yourself to work out. You have to train your coworkers, family, and friends to accept that you spend time getting in shape and it is one of your priorities. And yes, you will have to make some sacrifices.

Sometimes you may have to work out during an important sporting event or TV show. If it is so important then record it. You can't record your workouts. Sometimes you will have to give more time to your family on weekends you otherwise would have just spent relaxing. Working out is your time, but the people around you will discover that you will also be a better friend, employee, and family member once you have a better attitude and more energy. You may have to explain this fact to them at the beginning. You might have to shorten your lunch breaks a few times a week. Just do whatever you have to do to make it happen.

If you can manage five or even six days, then go for it, but you better be able to maintain it. If not, just go back down to four. The key thing to remember is that it must be doable in the long run. I can manage four days until I die, or five for a few months, or even six for a few weeks. Getting in shape doesn't happen overnight. All those BS 40-day programs are just that, BS. Plan for the long term, get the groundwork in place, and I promise you will succeed.

To complete the tasks in this book use the targets I provide. As you progress past those tasks you will learn to collect your own intelligence to determine your own targets. These targets will change as you improve but you need to start with the basics.

In the first Gulf War, we didn't initially destroy the Republican Guard army because there were too many threats defending them. First we had to "Degrade and Destroy the Air Defense System." During the first week of the war, the targeteers selected air defense nodes and command and control structures. After intelligence determined that air defense was effectively neutralized, the targeteers switched the primary targets to the real center of gravity: the Iraqi Republican Guard tank battalions.

A central tenet of this book is the requirement for accurate intelligence. Inaccurate intelligence was the main reason we went into Iraq the second time and lost thousands of American lives and hundreds of billions of taxpayer dollars. If we can't accurately measure our own progress, we will not have the correct intelligence to adjust our program. We will be making judgments based on incorrect information, which will most likely get in the way of reaching our objectives:

1. Work out at least four days a week.
2. Track workout data and weekly body composition.

The notes don't lie

I did my initial pilot training at Pensacola with the Navy. The plane was an old single propeller jet named the T-34. It has since been retired, but I can still imagine old Capt. Buras sitting behind me in the jet. I was in the front and he was in the back. He was a big, intimidating Mexican guy. He was rare in the Navy school since he was an Air Force fighter pilot. Most of the instructors were Navy helicopter pilots. Buras was much better than the Navy helicopter pilots and they seemed to know it. Probably because he'd told them he was better, but it was true.

He was my mentor and pointed out in cutting detail every mistake I made. He was good, dedicated, and I owe him for his hard work. I remember him telling me, "I shouldn't work harder than you," but I think he did. My mistakes were not insignificant: "Student called 'gen light out' when it was still on. 'RMI aligned' when it was 40 degrees off, and that he had avionics command when he did not. We don't read the checklist just to read it. If it looks like you will hit the GPU with your wing during the brake check, either correct or stop." He went on for a full page on my grade sheet.

"You don't graduate, your gradebook does," he said to me. With the amount of comments he wrote on all the grade sheets, it's a wonder I graduated. I have been graded like this on hundreds of upgrade sorties, by him and dozens of other instructors. It is painful but necessary.

In fact, it's unfortunate that after we become certified wingmen or flight leads, instructors don't keep grade sheets on us. The exceptional pilots tracked their own progress in a notebook or some other system. I took notes during debriefs and reviewed them later, but I would inevitably lose the sheet of paper. In the end I just took notes on the back of my flight card and then threw it away after a few months—what a mistake. The above-average pilots found a tracking system that worked for them.

If you find you aren't tracking your progress, figure out why you aren't tracking it and solve the problem. Get a smaller notebook. Maybe your phone works for you. Personally, I don't like using my phone but it doesn't matter what you decide as long as *it works*. You *must* find a system that works for you. I have a little notebook with a small pen that I keep in my gym bag. This works for me since I bring my gym bag home every night. If you don't, then use your brain to develop a different system that you will use in the long term.

Don't make it more difficult than it needs to be. Pick a workout program and write it in the notebook before you go to the gym. You only have to write the first week. Then you can just reference the past week for the program. While you're resting in between sets, write the weight and number of reps that you were able to do with good form. If you are focused on running or other cardio, then that is fine too: just write that in the book. The only gotcha is that the exercise has to be trackable. If you write "Jogged 20 min.," you won't know how far you jogged. Yeah, you'll remember for a few weeks, maybe a month, but then you'll forget. If you don't have accurate data, the wimpy voice will question your progress and hurt your motivation. It's good that you wrote *something*, but maybe you jogged a half mile at a kid's pace. Maybe you ran 3.5 miles at an Olympic runner's pace. You should write, "Jogged 20 min/2.2 miles." If you show this book to trainers or your mentor, they should be able to quickly understand your program and give you advice based on your progress. If you can track it you can manage it. Here is an example from my notebook from a random day last year:

June 23	(1.5 min. rest)
Deadlift	135x12, 185x12, 205x10, 8 *(new personal record!)*
Bench	135x10, 155x10, 165x7
Pull-ups	12, 9, 7 [superset with bench]
Handstand Push-ups	7, 7, 6
Row machine	120x10, 130x10, 130x9 [superset with handstand PU]
Jumped rope	30 sec (30 sec break) x 70 swings, 70, 70, 70, 70, 65, 70, 70 *Ran to and from gym* (approx. ¾ mile 7 min. each)

This is an advanced program since I am combining the upper body exercises together in supersets. It is a good technique to use to increase the intensity and shorten the time, but I don't recommend it at the beginning of a program. I don't write a bunch of extra information. Just what exercise, weight, and the number of reps. I wrote "1.5 minute rest," because that had changed from the previous week. 1-minute rest was too difficult for this program, so I increased it to 1.5 minutes. I don't note that the following day. This is the minimum amount of info we need to track. Start with the minimum and add as required.

The second necessary component you will track is body composition. People focus too much on body weight. Only when you combine bodyweight with waist measurements and your logbook can you find the truly important metric of body composition.

The scale tells your absolute weight change. The tape measure gives your fat increase or decrease, and the workout log indicates muscle increase or decrease (strength). Don't overstress your body weight. Like Yigit and I learned firsthand, the scale doesn't tell the complete story.

I recommend weighing yourself and measuring your waist once a week. Your body weight fluctuates throughout the day. If you drink 1 cup of water you weigh 1.4 lb. more. If you drink 1 liter of Gatorade you weigh 2.2 lb. more until your body processes the water.

On a side note, if you drink that liter of Gatorade before a 12-hour flight across the Atlantic Ocean in a fighter but didn't bring any piddle packs to urinate in, you will find yourself in a difficult situation. Having been in this situation I can tell you one viable solution that I tested, but don't fully endorse.

First I checked my helmet bag a sixth time and marveled at how I could have gotten in a single-seat airplane—knowing that I would have to fly 12 hours—without a bag to pee in. Then I held my pee for 3 hours and did not drink any liquids. After 3 hours I realized it would be physically impossible to hold it for another 9 hours and enacted my plan. I quickly drank the 1-liter bottle of Gatorade that I had in the tiny cockpit. I had to drink the entire bottle because I had already drunk an entire bottle of Gatorade. I needed a completely empty 1-liter receptacle to pee in. It worked but unfortunately I had 9 hours left to fly and no other bottles of Gatorade.

So, you see, you don't need to weigh yourself every day. If it helps your motivation to weigh yourself more often, do it. But keep in mind it's not an accurate measurement unless you check first thing in the morning. I might step on the scale a few times during the week but I only write down the number I get on Sunday before I eat or drink anything.

These are the primary targets. Work out at least four days a week and track your workout data and weekly body composition. If you hit these two targets you will get in shape. Let's look at some reasons why almost 80% of Americans don't do the recommended amount of exercise.[4]

---

[4] Ryan Jaslow, "CDC: 80 Percent of American Adults Don't Get Recommended Exercise," CBS News, May 3, 2013, http://www.cbsnews.com/news/cdc-80-percent-of-american-adults-dont-get-recommended-exercise/.

Chapter 6

Workout Threats

The biggest threats to your workout include lack of time, motivation, knowledge, money, or the idea that it's too late start. In air combat, the main threats are enemy fighters, surface-to-air missiles (SAMs) and guns, and incorrect intelligence. In a training exercise, after the mission commander has assigned the primary and secondary targets to the strikers, he normally has intel (the intelligence officer or team) go over the threats.

Intel stands up and briefs off a PowerPoint map projected onto a large screen. They start with the targets. They show some images and describe each target. The targets are represented by diamonds on the map. They then show slides of the enemy's first line of defense: the enemy airfields and combat air patrols. Intel explains what type of aircraft they expect and how many they can launch. They also indicate what weapons they are most likely to use and how proficient the pilots are.

The intel officer then covers the enemy's next line of defense: SAMs and guns (anti-aircraft artillery [AAA]). They brief the group on the last known location for the SAMs and AAA and show their threat rings on the map.

In every exercise, the first line of defense—and the most lethal threat to the good guys—is the enemy fighters. In modern combat, based on number of shoot downs, the SAMs and AAA are the most lethal. But in a real shooting war like the ones we train for, the fighters have to be dealt with or we will take huge losses.

A fighter is basically a fast-moving SAM. In WWII, our large bombers outflew the protection fighters, the P-38 and British Spitfire. Their small fuel tanks and short range required them to return to base early. Until the P-51 Mustang Fighter, with its extended range, entered the war, the bombers were left to defend themselves over enemy territory and thousands were shot down. Luftwaffe pilot Erich "Bubi" Hartmann shot down 352 Aircraft in WWII. Next was Barkhorn 301, Rall 275, Kittel 267, Nowotny 258, and so on and so forth. It's not until the 122nd pilot on the list, Juutilainen, with 94 kills, that the first non-Luftwaffe pilot emerges. (Go Finns!) But unfortunately, the next 30 pilots are Luftwaffe too, until a Japanese pilot comes along in these depressing statistics. The first American on the list is the 282nd— Richard Bong.

To combat the lethal enemy air forces, in all exercises I have been a part of, we send in the air-to-air fighters first. The wild weasels follow right behind them to suppress the SAMs and clear the way for the strikers. The air-to-air fighters are called offensive counter-air, or OCA (pronounced as initials). They sweep the enemy fighters out of the way by either shooting them or making them retreat. After the area is swept clear, the OCA fighters set up defensive combat air patrols near the targets. They defend against any new enemy fighters before they can shoot down our strikers (bombers).

While the enemy fighters are the first threat to be faced, in your fitness campaign, time is the first line of defense you need to confront. No time, not enough time, needing to make time…this is the wimpy voice and everyone's first excuse for not working out. I hate to break the news, but everyone in the world has the same amount of time. It's not like you have more time than I do. We each have 24 hours a day until we die. And of course we all have obligations to family, work, and ourselves.

When we say "I don't have enough time," we mean, "I can't make working out a priority right now because [insert lame excuse or excuses here]." The list has already been prepped by the wimpy voice before you even think it. It knows you are going to think about working out, and it already has the counterargument. It is inside your OODA loop.

Normally the wimpy voice says things like, "I can't wake up early and work out because I have to bring the kids to school; at work I can't get the time off because of this large project, and then after work I can't go because of some other excuse." The tactics I outline in the next section must first and foremost deal with the lack-of-time threat. With that dead weight lying in the road, we can't even begin the journey to getting in shape.

The second most dangerous threat in real combat is the SAMs, which are equivalent to lack of motivation in our fitness campaign. They are sneaky and hard as hell to kill. No matter what you do throughout your campaign (and your life) that sneaky punk lack of motivation will always be there. I have no doubt that every person deals with lack of motivation at some point. You can't destroy it, but if you can suppress this threat and hit the targets you will be successful.

There are some threats we can't destroy. But we can use tactics to suppress and neutralize them. Lack of motivation is one such threat. Indestructible threats may require us to change our plan but as long as we are open minded to all avenues of attack, we can avoid or suppress the threats on our way to the targets.

The third threat that can derail our plan is lack of assets. If we don't have enough bombs to destroy every target, do we cancel the mission? If there aren't enough air assets and our bombers will get slaughtered by the enemy air force, should we still push? These are real questions in a combat scenario, but in our campaign to get into great shape, the minimum assets required are much lower than you might think.

As I will explain in the tactics section, you don't need an expensive gym membership to get in shape. You don't even need access to weights. You can use body weight exercises. Although eating and drinking right is very important and supplements are a great advantage, you can reach your goals on any budget. You may have to make sacrifices such as eating out less, but you can still reach your goals on your current budget. Lack of assets, such as money or access to weight-lifting equipment, is not a valid threat and should not be a roadblock.

Lack of intelligence, on the other hand, is a dangerous threat. If what we think is correct is actually wrong, we will run our OODA loop from incorrect starting parameters. If we start from the wrong place we will not reach the target. Writing the workouts and body composition measurements down with adequate detail is important. Looking in the mirror and randomly weighing ourselves on a scale is not enough. We have to get accurate intel on how our body is reacting to the program.

You also must do the exercises correctly. My program has very few exercises because they are all compound exercises, which use a lot of muscles at the same time. If you have not done a lot of compound weight-lifting movements you will have to learn how to do them correctly. They are not difficult, but form is important to prevent injury and maximize results. You can reference my website www.chrislehto.com for short tutorials and pointers on doing the exercises correctly.

The final threat I would like to address is the idea that it's too late to start. Your wimpy voice may not use these exact words, but usually it sounds like "I'm too old" or "I'm too fat." This is wrong and just the wimpy voice ruining your plans again. It's never too late to start. There are thousands of examples of people who are older and fatter than you getting into fantastic shape.

Even Darth Vader changed—and he was the worst in the universe. All current scientific evidence shows that exercise improves quality and length of life when started at *any* age. I believe that older or fatter people have more incentive to work out because they will realize the largest gains and improvements in life.

Working out increases blood flow and has been proven effective against almost all types of disease including stroke, heart attack, and Alzheimer's. How many older people do you know who have broken bones in minor falls around the house? Weight lifting increases bone density and tendon and ligament strength. If you want to help your kids out in your old age, being in better shape will delay all the major diseases of our time, not to mention the day-to-day increase in strength and capability that you will enjoy. One recent study shows that losing 1 pound of belly fat was equivalent to taking 5 lb. of pressure off the knees. If you have knee pains, losing 5 lb. of belly fat will not only make you look and feel better, but it will also forever reduce 25 lb. of pressure on sensitive knees.

Most people think it is too late to start because they fear getting hurt. When my 67-year old parents started the program they were in rough shape. My father had just finished a year-long cancer recovery. My mother had ankle replacement surgery, a broken back, and could barely walk 20 yards. Weight lifting helped them prevent injury. As long as you sufficiently warm up and use proper form, the risk of injury from weight lifting is small. The benefits outweigh the risks.

Sometimes I get shoulder or elbow pains if I do certain exercises or if I push too hard and my form starts to degrade. If there is a slight pain I just avoid that exercise and take it easy for the next week on that part of my body. Maybe I take a rest week just to give my body a break. I just took a rest week because my right knee was complaining a little during squats. It wasn't painful or anything just a slight tingling. I corrected my form and leaned further back during the squat. Listen to your body while doing the exercises and don't overdo it.

Your muscles and joints shouldn't have sharp pains while you are lifting. If you are feeling a pain then just skip the exercise and do exercises that don't hurt. If nothing feels right take a few days off and see how you feel. But don't just quit. Stay on target.

Keep these threats in mind as you are doing the program. You will undoubtedly deal with lack of time, lack of motivation, and poor intelligence. Learn to identify them as threats when you encounter them. Use the tactics I outline in the next few chapters to avoid, suppress, or minimize them.

Tactics are the specific formations, weapons, timings, and techniques that we use to avoid the threats, hit the targets, and ultimately accomplish the task. Tactics make up the majority of a planning exercise. In my training exercise example, the general tactics dictate that the OCA jets will sweep the airspace clean of enemy fighters. They normally push (start the attack) into enemy territory supersonic in an offensive wall formation and launch long-range missiles against the enemy fighters. If the enemy fighters don't turn and run away they will be shot down. If they do turn around, our OCA fighters can take airspace from them. This is ideally how they sweep.

Normally, 5 minutes after the OCA assets push, the suppression of enemy air defense (SEAD; pronounced seed) assets push and start shooting pre-emptive suppression missile shots at the SAMs. The OCA and SEAD assets will set up defensive orbits and cover the target areas. They will defend the package of 20-30 strikers against the enemy fighters and SAMs. When the last bomb is dropped everyone gets out of dodge, with the OCA being the last ones out.

The OCA use their internal tactics to best sweep and defend the area. The SEAD use their own tactics to destroy or suppress the SAMs, and the strikers use their own internal tactics to best destroy the targets. This is the general plan, but something always forces the plan to change. Weather, aircraft malfunctions, or communication issues are examples of problems that can arise on our side. When a capable enemy force is added, anything can and usually does happen. It is up to the MC to adjust the mission real time so that there is a higher chance of success.

In American football, if the defense has an advantage at the start of a play, it is up to the offensive quarterback to assess the disadvantage to his team and change the play at the last second. In your own fitness campaign you are the mission commander. I will give the basic tactics, but when those tactics are not hitting the targets with enough accuracy, you must tweak the plan to ensure success.

The caveat is that the change must be simple to execute. Your body will adapt to any program. Your progress will undoubtedly slow at some point. Don't change the entire plan. Focus on the targets and make one change at a time and track the results. If you can't explain the change in two short sentences then it is too complicated.

The world is round

Everyone's workout intel is flawed. Yes this is a bold statement but hear me out. Try to find how many calories a squat "burns." Or *any* resistance exercise. The calories "burned" by our muscles are estimated using the Metabolic Equivalent of Task (MET). The MET is a unit of physical activity. But, and this is a big but, it is defined by how much oxygen you are using. Anaerobic processes don't use oxygen! They are anaerobic! When you lift a heavy weight you are using ATP and glycogen stores in your muscles. Just like bacteria. We are measuring the wrong damn thing.

This is the reason there are a million different exercise programs. No one knows how much energy your body uses during resistance training. Even though the Greeks learned that the earth was round over 2300 years ago, people still didn't believe it until the Middle Ages. It shouldn't be that hard. The moon is right there and it is a giant ball. The sun is shaped like a ball and reflects light on the moon. But when something gets into enough people's brains as truth, it becomes truth. And we wonder why our programs aren't working…the science is incomplete.

So what do we do about it? We do what they did thousands of years ago. If the model is incorrect just track what *is* correct. If you just count how many days it takes for spring to come every year and mark it on a signpost, you can plant crops. If you measure distances from one shore to another you don't need to know the earth is round to get to your destination. You just base your next action off of previously established data. Since the basic assumptions are incorrect we have to learn through trial and error.

Right now we are using the BS calorie-burning system. Cardio is one way to lose fat but it is a very inefficient and time-consuming way to do it. From my personal experience weight resistance training caused my body to lose fat fast. I know this because I tracked the program and watched it happen.

Watch any of the big names on YouTube. I like Brandon Carter at www.highlifeworkout.com, Mike Chang at www.sixpackshortcuts.com, and Chris Jones at beastmodejonescoaching.com. They are all ripped and do relatively little cardio. If Carter and Chang do any cardio at all, it is only after a strength training workout. They learned through trial and error what works. They are excellent references and have their own styles that you may like.

I suspect most fitness models do resistance training. Why? Because resistance training uses *way more* energy than cardio in a smaller amount of time. The simple reason is the ATP and glycogen stores of the muscles are used by anaerobic processes which are 15 times less efficient than the aerobic process.

Chapter 7

Workout Program

Here is our big picture plan to avoid the threats and hit our two primary targets: work out at least four days a week and track workout data and weekly body composition.

Big Picture Plan: Get Started

Buy or steal a small notebook and pen,
Choose a workout program,
I recommend compound exercises for 25 minutes:
- *1 min. rest in between sets*
- *8 min. of HIIT cardio or 15 min. of steady-state cardio at the end*

Write the program in the notebook,
Find a venue and do the program (at home, a park, or a gym),
Write down weight and reps for each set (with good form) in the notebook,
Write down cardio parameters (how many miles run, mountain climbers accomplished, etc…),
Once a week, in the morning, write down weight and waist measurements,
Accomplish for 1 month.

To prepare for working out get all your equipment ready the day prior. Don't give the wimpy voice any leeway to make excuses. Put shoes, shorts, socks, shirt and underwear in a bag. If you are going to shower somewhere else bring a towel, sandals, and some soap. Put the notebook in the bag. If there is no water at the venue then put a bottle of water in the bag also. If you use supplements put them in your bag. Put the bag next to the front door so you won't forget it. Then the next day just go to wherever you need to go and do the workout.

Just pick a program

People spend too much mental effort choosing a program. There is even exercise snobbery. I was doing P90X and some friends gave me a hard time since that was old and the new Insanity program "works much better." I did both programs and saw results with both. I believe heavier resistance training is more effective for me, but I was in better shape after completing both P90X and Insanity.

The problem with doing specific 30-day programs is that the goal is to just finish the program. Just like the marathoners, once you finish the program your willpower will dwindle and it will be difficult to continue. Keep it simple and do the program I recommend. You don't need to waste mental energy trying to choose a program. Track the workouts and note your progress. If you don't like the results, change the program. But continue to track your workouts. Seeing progress on paper will keep you invested in the long term. I will describe the workout first and then explain using personal experience and scientific evidence why I think it is the most effective.

If you can only do three days instead of four, then just start with three days! Don't quit because four is too many. After a while you can work up to four and then when you are comfortable doing four days a week for a month you have completed Task 1. Then you can move to five and maybe even six workouts a week if you enjoy it.

After I select how many days a week I can work out, I build the program. For a 3-day program I would do full-body weight workouts. On two of those days, I would also do cardio and on the other day I would work the stomach instead of cardio. If I can work out four days, which I recommend, then I would still do full body workouts but I would alternate the focus every other day: upper body, lower body, upper body, lower body.

After a few months I switch up the workouts. Everyone is different. What works for you won't necessarily work for me. Your notebook will tell you what program gets you the best results. For each program, do 3 sets of each exercise (8-12 reps). If that feels easy, try four sets. No matter which program you pick, definitely stick with compound movements as much as possible. Compound movements get you the most bang for your workout buck. They use way more muscles than isolation exercises. The more muscles you use the more energy you use. You will lose more fat and gain more muscle in the same amount of time.

Two 4-day programs for the gym

Program 1: Upper/Lower Body Split

Splitting upper and lower body parts onto separate days allows two days of rest before working the same muscle group again.

Always:	Start with a 5 minute warm-up on the treadmill/elliptical; stretch 5 min.; 3 sets of 8-12 reps all exercises.
Monday:	Bench Press, Military press, Lat pull-downs, Back rows, Cardio (HIIT 8 min. or steady-state 15 min.)
Tuesday	Squats, Leg extensions, Leg curls/calves HIIT abdominal cardio (mountain climbers or crunches) 8 min.
Wednesday:	*Rest*
Thursday:	Incline bench press, Bench press, Back rows, Lateral raises Cardio (HIIT 8 min. or steady-state 15 min.)
Friday:	Deadlifts, Lunges/calves, Incline sit-ups and leg raises Cardio (HIIT 8 min. or steady-state 15 min.)

Move the days around as you see fit to match your energy level and schedule. I also change the days periodically to keep the workout interesting.

Program 2: Full Body

I've found my body reacts better to full body workouts. They are more intense than splits so I recommend one day of only cardio combined with abdominal work as a break for the muscles. Use full body if you want to lose fat faster and want a tougher workout. If it's too difficult, lower the weight or switch to upper/lower split.

Each workout day:	Start with a 5 min warm-up on the treadmill/elliptical; stretch 5 min.; 3 sets of 8-12 reps all exercises.
Monday:	Squats, Bench Press, Military press, Lat pull-downs (pull-ups), Cardio (HIIT 8 min. or steady-state 15 min.).
Tuesday	HIIT abdominal cardio 8 min., Steady-state cardio 25 min..
Wednesday:	Deadlifts, Incline bench press, Back rows, Lunges/calves, Cardio (HIIT 8 min. or steady-state 15 min.).
Thursday:	*Rest.*
Friday:	Same as Monday.

Change the days in the second week, for example: deadlift on Monday and Friday and do squats.

Two 4-Day programs for body weight exercises

The one caveat for body weight exercises is that you need to invest in a pull-up bar. Unless you have heavy weights at home (to do bent-over rows) it is difficult to work your back effectively. I bought the Iron Gym Total Upper Body Workout bar for $36. You slide it over a door jam and it works great. With that one piece of equipment you can get a reasonable total body workout at home. If the exercises are too easy, make them more challenging by wearing a backpack filled with bags of rice.

You can get in shape doing this workout, but to continue to strengthen your lower back you will need to do deadlifts and squats with weights too. Once you gain strength, a backpack will probably not be enough. Keep an open mind and cross that bridge when you reach it.

Program 1: Upper/Lower Body Split

This program provides more rest in between working different muscle groups. You work each muscle group twice a week instead of three times in the full-body program. Easier versions of each exercise are inside parenthesis.

Always:	5-min. warm-up (run in place/jumping jacks, 5 min. stretch, 3 sets of max reps).
Monday:	Push-ups (knee push-ups), Pull-ups (hold and hang for time), Handstand push-ups (jack-knife push-ups), Dips off a chair or the Iron Gym, Cardio (HIIT if inside 8 min., or Steady-state if outside [run, bike, swim, etc.] 15 min.).
Tuesday	One-legged squats (normal squats), Lunges (in between chair lunges), Single leg calf raises off a stair (two-leg calf raises off a stair), HIIT abdominal cardio.
Wednesday:	*Rest.*
Thursday:	Same as Monday.
Friday:	Same as Tuesday.

Program 2: Body Weight (Full Body)	
Monday:	Push-ups (knee push-ups), Pull-ups (hold and hang for time), Handstand push-ups (jack-knife push-ups), One-legged squats (Body Squats), Single leg calf raise on stair (two-leg calf raise on stair), Cardio (HIIT if inside 8 min., or Steady-state if outside [run, bike, swim, etc.] 15 min.).
Tuesday (or Thursday)	HIIT abdominal cardio, Cardio (HIIT if inside 12 min., or Steady-state if outside [run, bike, swim, etc.] 25 min.).
Wednesday:	Push-ups (knee push-ups), Pull-ups (hold and hang for time), Handstand push-ups (jack-knife push-ups), Lunges, HIIT abdominal.
Friday:	Same as Monday.

The following week, switch the days to keep your body guessing and to keep the workouts fresh. If you have weights at home, then add compound weight movements as required. Reference the gym workout as a guide. Pick the plan you want to continue working with. If you don't like this program, just pick a different one! But do it and remember to write everything down.

I change my program slightly every few months to keep my workouts interesting and my body constantly adapting. I ensure I do compound movements but I might add a different exercise or use a different machine. Anytime you switch even a small variable such as the grip of your pull-ups, your body will react differently. On Monday do regular pull-ups. Then when you have to do them again do chin ups. This small change will work different muscles in your body.

If I do change my workouts, after a few months I return to the basic lifts of bench, pull-ups, squats, and deadlifts to judge my progress. This way I can tell if the change was beneficial or not.

If your form breaks down before you complete 8 reps then the exercise is too difficult. Just do an easier modified version of it until you get stronger. Moving from knee push-ups to regular push-ups is a marked increase in capability. Being able to do your first handstand push-up is a very motivating experience. I remember my first muscle-up and handstand push-up. Stay on track and I promise that one day you will be able to do the activity you dream of doing. Mehmet just gave up too soon.

To gym or not to gym

If you have access to a gym, you should use it. If you don't, then do body weight workouts at home or at a park. Although body weight workouts can work well, I've found that resistance training with free weights or on weight machines adds flexibility to a program. As Mehmet learned, he was too weak to do push-ups and too embarrassed to do knee push-ups. Those were his two options. If he had had access to some dumbbells, he could have done bench presses for a few weeks until he was strong enough to do real push-ups. Personally I don't see any difference between pressing light weight dumbbells and doing knee push-ups but it was a critical factor in his brain.

Using free weights allows you to increase the resistance one pound at a time. This is how those strong guys and girls you see in the gym got so strong. Every time they worked out they maximized to within a pound of what their body could do. Every workout they got a smidgen stronger. As long as a reasonable diet is in place your body has no option but to improve; in fact, it is *impossible* for it not to.

Be persistent and creative in executing your program

A fighter pilot without a pencil is like a knight without a sword. It's okay if you only have a pen, but the assumption widely held among fighter pilots is you will find a pencil as soon as possible. We have to write down critical information such as friendly coordinate locations or enemy positions. A pencil is better than a pen because we make mistakes and need to correct the mistake as cleanly as possible to avoid confusion. If you don't have either, you might as well not even call yourself a fighter pilot. I would *never* ask to borrow a pen or pencil unless it is from a close friend in the squadron. Of course I've found myself in the cockpit without a pencil and it is a horrible feeling.

In Korea one of my favorite squadron commanders lost a pencil in the cockpit. Not only did he not have a pencil but he had dropped a foreign object in the jet. The jet couldn't fly until the pencil was found. This is a double faux-pas. The crew chief spent 30 minutes looking for the pencil until he finally found it. The next day the commander had his pencil tied by a string to his checklist. He was an amazing pilot and leader. We all make mistakes, but the successful people identify the problem and fix it. Do the same in your workout plans. If something isn't working for you just find the solution and move on.

Chapter 8

Minimize Time over Target with 4 Tactics

Combating the lack-of-time threat

The first and most difficult obstacle to overcome in starting any workout program is lack of time. Lack of time is equivalent to the air-to-air defense fighter in the examples above. If you don't account for it you will be shot down before you get to the target. What we are really saying when we say we don't have time is that we can't make working out a priority because other things in life are more important. We all have the same 24 hours in a day. Those people you see who are in fantastic shape aren't wizards. They don't manipulate space-time to work full-time jobs with kids and still get in a workout. They just devote their time to investing in their health. Like I argued earlier, what in life could possibly be more important than your body? You want to help your kids? It will be a whole lot easier with 30% more energy. You have to work long hours? Being in shape gives you mental and physical energy to be more productive at work.

And when I say that people in great shape use their time smarter, I don't mean they schedule every minute of their day. But, they do replace unproductive activities with activities that invest in the future. They put their time towards an energy-producing asset—a healthy body—instead of energy-consuming activities like most of the useless stuff we do in our free time.

Make time for working out

My first suggestion is to try and work out as part of your normal work schedule. Most of us work five days a week. If you can work out on four out of five of those days you will complete the task. Personally I've found that if I can replace unproductive time at work with productive time, I can "make" time to work out. It's not possible to work 8-10 hours straight without taking mental breaks. I recommend breaks. Your brain needs them. But keep them short and then get back to work. It is very easy for mental breaks to extend longer and longer until we are actually wasting time. Everyone is guilty in this regard, including me.

The difference is now that working out is a priority for me, when I find myself not working I put myself back to work. If I need a mental break I take it, but after a few minutes I work to get stuff done. This way my productivity remains the same even if I devote an hour and 15 minutes of my work day to fitness. I also sometimes get home 30 minutes later or leave 30 minutes earlier in the morning.

To replace less productive, potential time-wasting activities with health-promoting activities, I tracked my time: 10 minutes searching the internet, 10 minutes reading a magazine, 20 minutes talking with friends, and 20 minutes checking email. I replaced it with one hour of working out. You only have to do it four days a week.

Not every person can squeeze a workout into a busy day, but if your office has a gym or there's one just around the corner, see if you can make it happen with some creative planning. Shift a few less important tasks around or postpone them. If you can't find the time to work out during your work hours, then you will have to work out in your free time. I think this is a last resort, but do what you need to do. If you work out Saturday and Sunday, then you should be able to find time to work out and take a shower twice during the work week. However you do it, make 75 minutes available four times a week.

Time-saving tactic 1: compound movements

In order to maximize our results in the minimum amount of time we will use four techniques. The first and, I believe, most important technique is to use compound exercises. A compound exercise is one that requires two joints to execute. An isolation exercise only requires one joint. For example during a push-up your elbow joints bend and your shoulder joints rotate. Both joints are required for the exercise. But during a bicep curl, only your elbow joint bends. The shoulder joint remains stationary. The push-up is a compound exercise and the bicep curl is an isolation exercise.

By using two joints you use many more muscles. As an example, if you are doing an isolation exercise such as the bicep curl, you are working your two bicep muscles (brachii and brachialis), the deltoids in your shoulders, and several wrist extensor muscles in your forearm. Sounds like a lot right?

Now compare that amount to the number of muscles worked in a pull-up. In the pull-up exercise (called lat pull-downs if done on a machine), you work the same muscles already mentioned in the bicep curl *and* the large back muscles such as the latissimus dorsi, infraspinatus, lower trapezius, erector spinae, and external oblique. Plus, depending on your grip, you also work your pectoralis chest muscles and the long tricep muscle.

By doing pull-ups instead of bicep curls *in the same amount* of time, you work additional large muscles in your body *and* your biceps. There are hundreds of compound exercises but the exercises that I will focus on are pull-ups, back rows, deadlifts, military press, squats, and lunges.

Compound exercises also use more of your cardiovascular system. In the same amount of time in the gym, you use more energy and gain more health benefits if you replace isolation exercises with compound exercises. You will strengthen more nerves, ligaments, and tendons. Plus, for the following 48 hours, more of your muscles will be using energy to repair themselves. In the same amount of time you will gain more muscle and lose more fat. This is what I mean by working smarter. You are maximizing your results based on a time limitation. Everyone in the world has some sort of time limitation. Don't just quit because you don't have enough time, determine how to maximize the time you do have.

Time-saving tactic 2: Check a clock in between sets

Another key technique to maximize our time-effectiveness while working out is to limit rest between sets. I recommend a rest time of 1 to 1.5 minutes. Actually keep track during the workout using a clock, watch, or phone. If you want to focus more on cardio or need to shorten your workout, the first step is to lower your rest time to 1 minute. If that makes your workout too long, go to 45 or even 30 seconds. Personally, I like 1 minute for upper body exercises and 1.5 minutes if I am doing lower body lifts or supersetting upper body (which I do consistently now).

One thing to remember when shortening your rest times is that you won't be able to lift the same amount of weight. With shorter rest times your muscles and cardiovascular system will be more fatigued. This seems obvious but I have felt demotivated by my strength "going down" when actually my shortened rest times were the culprit. If you can lift the same amount of weight in a shorter rest time then you have become stronger. Also, if you can lift the same amount of weight and your body weight has gone down, you have become stronger. Generally, if you give your body more rest you will be able to lift more weight for more reps.

Time-saving tactic 3: Do three sets

For these workouts I recommend doing 3 sets of each exercise. The scientific reason is explained as follows in the excellent book *Nutrient Timing*: "one set of ten bicep curls results in 12 percent loss of muscle glycogen; three sets result in 35 percent depletion, and six sets result in 40 percent depletion".[5] You would have to do twice the work just to go from 35% depletion to 40% depletion. Based on this data, assuming approximately 10 reps in each set, 3 sets maximizes your results in relation to time.

The non-scientific reason that I recommend 3 sets is that for these workouts, normally 3 working sets is enough for me, especially if I superset. If you do not feel adequately worked then by all means do 4 sets or superset the upper body exercises.

Time-saving tactic 4: HIIT cardio takes less time

The final technique I use to shorten my workout time is high-intensity interval training or HIIT cardio. All it means is that you work out at a high intensity for a short time (10-60secs) followed by a short rest (10-60secs). This is one "rep" and we repeat this in intervals, thus the name HIIT. Sprinting is a type of HIIT cardio, but it can be done with any exercise. I like mountain climbers for abdominal work. It is more fun than sit-ups and it works my cardiovascular system.

The other option for cardio is moderate-intensity continuous training or steady-state cardio. This is the normal cardio we all know and love: jogging, biking, swimming, elliptical machine, etc. Your heart rate stays roughly the same, in a steady state, in this type of cardio.

The way I incorporate HIIT is to do 8 minutes of interval training after my weight lifting. The actual exercise is not that important. Again, anything can work. Running in place, jumping jacks, jumping rope, burpees, or working on an elliptical machine,

---

[5] John Ivy and Robert Portman, *Nutrient Timing: The Future of Sports Nutrition* (Laguna Beach, CA: Basic Health Publications, 2004), 34.

stair stepper, or bike are a few examples. The important part is that your heart rate stays high and it is difficult to talk during high-intensity sections. HIIT cardio is difficult, but it is over fast.

If my shoulders aren't feeling 100% then I jog for 1 minute and sprint for 15 seconds. If my shoulders feel good then I do 30 seconds of burpees with 30 seconds of rest. If I am bored of both of those then I jump rope for 30 seconds and rest for 30 seconds. I have an app on my phone that times intervals. I use it for rowing machines and mountain climbers. It really doesn't matter what exercise you do as long as you are working hard for a short time (at the maximum effort you can muster) and then resting for a short time. The best part is that it's over quickly and it's fun because you can mix up your cardio workouts with many different options. To learn more about these exercises, see www.chrislehto.com.

Is HIIT better than steady-state cardio?

There are many studies that have found HIIT to be more effective than steady-state cardio at decreasing certain markers for cardiovascular disease. As an example, according to one recent study, HIIT cardio was more effective than steady-state training at lowering pulse wave reflection, an established marker associated with arterial stiffness and cardiovascular disease. [6] HIIT cardio was also found to be more effective than steady-state cardio at improving O2 pulse curves, a marker of cardio respiratory fitness.[7]

But as effective as HIIT cardio may be at increasing cardio respiratory markers, there are also studies that suggest it is actually not more effective than steady-state cardio for respiratory fitness. For instance, one study found that "it remains

---

[6] H. Hanssen et al., "Acute effects of interval versus continuous endurance training on pulse wave reflection in healthy young men," *Atherosclerosis* 238, no. 2 (2015), http://www.ncbi.nlm.nih.gov/pubmed/25558034.

[7] G.C. Cardozo, R.B. Oliveira and P.T. Farinatti,"Effects of high intensity interval versus moderate continuous training on markers of ventilator and cardiac efficiency in coronary heart disease patients," *Scientific World Journal* (2015), http://www.ncbi.nlm.nih.gov/pubmed/25741531.

'unclear' whether [HIIT cardio] elicits a superior improvement in cardiorespiratory fitness relative to [steady-state cardio].[8]

The results are somewhat contested but I believe the benefit of HIIT cardio is that it depletes glycogen stores in the muscles much *faster* than steady-state cardio. Since HIIT uses close to maximum muscle force, the body must use anaerobic energy processes. If you have already done a difficult, glycogen-depleting resistance workout such as the program I recommend, doing HIIT cardio will not give you much advantage. What I find to be the biggest advantage of HIIT cardio is that it takes less time and I can combine it with different workouts. I feel like I get the same amount of cardio in half the time. Lately I have been doing steady-state cardio and I am also getting good results. Mix it up to keep your workouts interesting. Cheat to win.

Combating loss of motivation

What affects your motivation? Why do you personally not work out? I'm more likely to skip a workout if I don't schedule it in the morning. The day gets busier, I get more and more tired, and my motivation wanes. In order to avoid this threat, I work out first thing in the morning. As soon as I can get 1.5 hours of non-scheduled time available, I drop everything I am doing and go to the gym. If I wait until after lunch, the chances are higher something important will come up and interfere with my plans.

In my fitness analogy, fighting surface-to-air missiles (SAMs) is very similar to fighting a decrease in motivation. Whether in combat or during a training exercise, the next most dangerous threat after the enemy fighter is the SAM network. These are large, capable, ground-based systems that often can move on a tank or wheel chassis. They are dangerous and sneaky. A Russian SA-6 shot down the famous F-117 Stealth Fighter in Serbia. They

---

[8] B.H. Roxburgh et al., "Is moderate intensity exercise training combined with high intensity interval training more effective at improving cardiorespiratory fitness than moderate intensity exercise training alone?" *Journal of Sports Science and Medicine* 13, no. 3 (2014):702-7. http://www.ncbi.nlm.nih.gov/pubmed/25177202.

are lethal and if there are several of them working together they can be very dangerous.

The US military developed Wild Weasel squadrons during Vietnam to specifically target and suppress the enemy SAMs. One key point in fighting SAMs is that even though we want to destroy them, if we can just suppress them and still hit the targets, then we have completed the task. If a boxer wins a match by TKO he still wins, right? What the Air Force has learned about SAMs is that those bastards can be hard to kill. They move and hide in the trees and only transmit their signals for short periods of time when they need guidance. They are controlled by humans, and humans are sneaky.

For the Stinkbug (F-117) shoot-down, the wily Serbians knew the return route of the fighters. They came down a valley on predictable schedules. The Serbians did the calculations and fired the missile in the general direction of the next incoming fighter. This time they got lucky and hit a Stealth F-117. It may be stealth, but it still exists in the real world and a lucky shot is always possible.

The easiest and safest way to not get shot down by a SAM system is to avoid it. If you know where it is, don't go close enough for it to shoot you. We plot the effective ranges of the known SAMs and plan our route around them.

Pretty simple, right? Well, first you have to know where they are and you have to know how far they can shoot. We rely on intelligence and other experienced Wild Weasel fighter pilots for this info. Since you won't have a team of professionals to get you intel—and most of the nutrition and exercise info is wrong anyway—you will have to figure it out yourself.

If you don't work out one day, don't get angry or lose heart. Just find out why you didn't go and fix the problem. If you lose your motivation every time you go to the bar. Guess what? Avoid the bar. Schedule your off days so you can go to the bar without it affecting your workout schedule. Plan a different route.

If you always meet friends at the bar, try to set up a different activity. If you go to the bar anyway, then just drink water or tea.

If your friends don't understand or support your choices, then how good of friends are they anyway? Don't get emotional. Use the OODA loop: observe why you didn't go to the gym, orient by looking at options to fix the problem, decide on a new game plan, and act on the new game plan. Then use the loop again. Did it fix the problem? That's it. That's all you have to do. Don't overcomplicate it. Just hit the targets week in and week out. KISS.

Chapter 9

Avoid (or Suppress) the Threats and Hit the Targets

Let's say you can't avoid the threat so your only option is to suppress it. You have to go to the ice cream parlor twice a week for some reason and they always have your favorite dessert. In suppression of enemy air defense (SEAD) tactics there are two basic types of suppression. The first is pre-emptive missile attack and the second is reactive missile attack. Generally we employ both.

We shoot pre-emptive radar-seeking missiles before we enter the threat ring. This makes the surface-to-air missiles (SAMs) shut off their radars so they can't attack us. Then our suppression of enemy air defense (SEAD) assets wait and shoot reactive shots at any enemy radars that turn on. Reactive shots are more difficult to execute but sometimes, we do what we have to do. For instance, if we are blindsided by a pop-up missile system in the target area then we have to defend with a reactive shot. Or if the enemy is able to move their mobile assets to a different location we have to be prepared for the chance that the mobile SAM will come online.

In our ice cream parlor example, how can we suppress the threat of just sitting around drinking and eating junk food? For pre-emptive shots, I like to drink a protein shake before I go to tempting restaurants or bars. Most restaurant food is unhealthy, consisting mostly of fast-digesting carbohydrates. By filling up on a protein shake before I get there, I can still enjoy a little of the carbs but I am not really hungry for them. If you put other fats like coconut oil or peanut butter in your shake you will be more satiated and have the energy to just sit around and talk for hours. If I am already full it is much easier to just have a taste of the junk food instead of eating a lot of it. Sometimes I will also alter my food plan during the day to offset any junk food I might be forced to eat that night.

If we can't use pre-emptive shots, then we have to suppress using reactive shots. If it is getting harder and harder to say no to certain foods or drinks, the easiest way to survive is to compress the time over target. If we are in the threat zone for the minimum amount of time, the enemy has less time to attack us. So just leave earlier. You can still go to the event or party, and you can still have a good time, but there really is no reason to sit around for 5 hours. Leave after 2 or 3 hours. You will be amazed how much more you can accomplish and how much better you will feel. And the best part is you still get to enjoy your normal activities. You just moderate them and suppress the threat.

Focus on the targets and don't let anyone interfere

The key to being successful at suppressing and avoiding threats is to make the task and the targets a priority. You will still spend time with your family and friends but hitting your targets is always in the back of your mind. If you explain this to your friends after a while they will support you if they are really your friends. Don't be surprised or upset if they don't support you in the beginning and haven't yet realized you are serious. Most likely, they won't fully support you. Pop-up threats to your motivation can appear where you least expect them. I told a few family members of my goal to write a book and their initial gut response was "don't quit your day job." When I quit drinking I lost a few friends, apparently because we were only connected through drinking.

If you decide to change your life, you will find that people will not be excited about it at first. I believe deep down they feel they should also change and when you change this puts pressure on them. It sounds ridiculous, but it's true. They feel threatened that you are making positive changes. The wimpy voice in their head starts blaming you and your crazy ideas for making them feel guilty or bad about themselves. So instead of being happy for you and supporting you, many times unfortunately, these people can subconsciously hope you fail or even sabotage your plans. It is not their fault, it is just human nature. No one wants to change. We understand and are comfortable with the status quo. Changing the status quo requires energy and a route into the unknown. Many times we would rather be unhappy in a familiar situation than venture into difficult and unfamiliar territory.

If you don't have to explain your goal to anyone, then don't do it. I've found the best way to reach a goal is to just reach it on my own with the support of my immediate family and maybe a few friends. Your friends aren't going to really help you reach your fitness goal. A workout buddy can help you reach your goal a little faster, but you'll be dependent on someone else. If they are really dedicated to getting in shape then they can be a powerful asset. But truly, the only thing between you now and you in the best shape of your life is you.

In my experience, friends can help by just not giving me a hard time about my priorities and being happy for me when I do reach my goals. If your friends want to spend time with you they can hang out with you while you work out or they can work around your schedule priorities.

Motivation is a long-term proposition

We all have motivation in the beginning right? It's easy to be on-guard and on-point at the beginning of the war. But what about the hundredth day? What about when "life happens" and it gets difficult? Maybe your workout buddy lost their will and quit. Maybe your girlfriend, boyfriend, or spouse left you, or maybe you lost your job. What about when you get sick? How do we continue to suppress lack of motivation and continue to the target day-in and day-out?

The biggest motivator in the long term is PROGRESS. This is why tracking your progress is so important. When we see progress towards a goal, it motivates us to continue and work even harder. This is one reason why CrossFit is so successful. CrossFitters track their progress and write it up on the board in their gym for everyone to see. Seeing this progress and having their friends excited about it is what drives motivation. The other reason I believe CrossFit is successful is that it uses compound exercises. I personally don't do CrossFit, but if it works for you then go for it. I did it several years ago and kept getting injured. It was at the beginning of CrossFit and I didn't have a coach so maybe one day I will give it another shot. For now, I like my own program.

When you are loading a computer program and the little progress bar completely stops, how does it feel? Or how about when the time-to-complete actually increases? It's demoralizing and that's only 5-10 minutes of our time.

But when the progress bar continues in one smooth motion—it may take twice as long—but we are content to watch it until the end. It may take an hour, but I know when it will end. It is making progress. Yet when it just stops on 16%, who knows how long it will take to finish.

If you track your progress, you will at least have a progress bar. Even if you are seeing no progress, you will still know without a doubt that you aren't getting worse. The task isn't increasing in time. If you follow the plan I outline you will see progress. And that is all we need to feed the fire of our motivation for the long term. Once we see a little progress and our bodies are used to the program, we can ramp it up a little bit. Once we see a little more progress, we continue to slowly tighten the screws. Increasing progress creates motivation which creates more progress. Soon enough, we have reached our task and can move on to the next task. Track your progress and refer back to it for motivation. Tracking not only guides your program, it drives it.

Lack of assets (money)

If you believe money is a threat then you are thinking about it the wrong way. First use what you have. If you can't afford a gym membership or don't have access to a weight room then do body weight exercises. You can do body weight exercises for a long time before you hit a plateau. Depending on your goals you may never need to go to a gym. Put some books or water bottles in a back pack for weight and all of a sudden you have weighted push-ups, pull-ups, squats, and lunges. Throw in some shoulder exercises and sit-ups and you can work your whole body. That is actually enough to get into great shape.

The other benefit of body weight exercises is that you have the option to do them wherever you want. Since all you need is your body and a little bit of space, the workout is extremely flexible. On nice sunny days you can work out outside in the park. When you are traveling you can work out in the crappy hotel gym with body weight exercises without a problem. If they don't have a crappy hotel gym you can work out in your hotel room.

However if you have access to at least some money, I recommend thinking of your body as a multi-million dollar fighter jet. You can fly the best fighter aircraft in the world, but if you don't spend money on working missiles you are going to lose. You should invest money to maximize your return. A longer and healthier life is an amazing return on investment. I bet you will spend more on your car next year in insurance and payments than you will spend following the basic plan in this book. Your body is your most valuable asset and yet healthy food, supplements, and gym memberships are "too expensive." You don't necessarily need those things to achieve the body you want. Theoretically you can get into amazing shape without healthy food or supplements, but it will definitely take longer.

Combating a lack of accurate and timely intel

Form is sometimes important in life and sometimes it isn't. Back in 2006, I deployed with my squadron to Balad Air Base in Iraq. It's a giant air base located 25 miles northeast of Baghdad. We took the base over from Saddam. Its central location allowed us to take off and reach most of Iraq quickly. It was also the largest concentration of foreign troops, so the base was consistently mortared 2-3 times a week. Prior to the base getting the Iron Dome gun defense system, the rockets and mortars just landed on the base. At my initial in-processing brief after unloading from the C-17 onto the hot tarmac, the female airman said "as long as you don't hear 'incoming' from the speaker system the mortars are landing somewhere else on the base." We still needed to take cover when we heard the normal sirens but the mortars weren't landing in our sector.

We settled into day-to-day ops working 12 hour shifts flying or sitting duties at work and then working out, watching movies, playing ping pong or video games, and taking classes in our time off. We would hear the distant boom of the mortars and, wherever we were, take cover behind sandbags for about 30 minutes until the all clear came. After a few months, it became routine. The scariest part was when Explosive Ordnance Disposal teams would destroy captured weapons near our sleeping huts. For some reason they never let us know in advance and just scared the hell out of us with the large explosions.

I only heard "incoming" once in five months at the base. That day a good buddy of mine, Stevo, and I were walking to the field hospital. He had wanted to help carry the wounded soldiers from the field hospital on base and load them on the C-17s bound for Europe. I had the day off so I went with him. We were in our Air Force workout gear of shorts and a t-shirt. The threat level mandated that we wear our body armor but we could strap our helmets to our belts. The heavy Kevlar helmets were uncomfortable to wear for long periods of time so everyone strapped them to the body armor vest. The problem was my helmet strap had broken. Rather than go through the hassle to find out how to replace the helmet or fix the strap, I had poor form and just wore my helmet with the strap hanging down.

It was hot that day and the walk to the field hospital was a mile walk along a dusty dirt road. We were sweating and I complained about having to wear my helmet.

"Why don't you just get your helmet fixed then?" Stevo asked and mockingly pointed to his helmet swinging from his belt.

"Well Stevo, in case you haven't noticed we are in a combat zone," I pointed to my helmet on my head in the same mocking gesture. I think I was just young and lazy.

Then from a hidden speaker right next to us, a clear calm voice that I will never forget called "incoming…incoming." We both looked wide-eyed at each other.

"JUMP IN THE DITCH!" I yelled and pointed to the side of the road.

We dove into the ditch. The problem is in the desert of Iraq there is no water. If there is no water there is no need for a real ditch. So we laid down in the 1-inch deep indentation in the dirt and tried to hunker down. Luckily for me, my helmet was already on! The first mortar hit about 70 meters away on the tarmac next to us and made a loud explosion. They always attacked in waves, so we waited a few seconds for the next rounds to hit. I looked up to see Stevo fiddling with his helmet strap. Lying face down in the dirt with mortar rounds going off nearby is a difficult time to undo a finicky helmet strap.

I pointed and laughed "HAH! I told you!" and then got my head down again as the other rounds hit about 10 meters closer. Although Stevo didn't think it was too funny at the time, he did laugh about it later. The mortar shrapnel damaged a C-130 cargo plane sitting on the tarmac but no one was injured, thankfully.

That day, poor form in maintaining uniform adherence gave me the last laugh, but in the action of working out and lifting weights, good form is extremely important. Having good form when we do exercises limits our exposure to injury. It also allows us to objectively track our progress so we don't overtax our bodies. Good form maximizes tension on the muscle while minimizing stress on our joints and ligaments. We always maximize gains and minimize chance for injury.

Learn to use proper form and stop lifting when form degrades

Proper form is important for two reasons. First, it limits momentum in our lifts and decreases the chance that we will overstress muscles and ligaments. Think of lifting a heavy box off the ground with your back curved. Second, proper form makes tracking our progress easier and clearer.

Experienced weight lifters can cheat and still make the exercise work, but they know what they are doing. They won't count those cheat reps as actual reps. Those are just bonus reps to fatigue the muscle. If I am doing pull-ups and on my tenth pull-up I push off the ground to get my chin to the bar, I don't count that pull-up. I write 9 pull-ups on my sheet. The last pull-up was a cheat rep. These can be dangerous because we do cheat reps when our muscles are fatigued. We also engage other support muscles. When I cheat doing a pull-up and push off the ground I am using my calves and legs, not the targeted muscles of a pull-up. A clearer example is military press or handstand push-ups. If we cheat while pushing heavy weight above our head, we risk injuring our neck or back.

If you can't do a full extension pull-up, then by all means cheat until you can do one by not going all the way down or using a box or something else. But you need to know that when you use bad form, you can introduce momentum into the exercise. The momentum can knock you off balance and overstretch muscles. If you are letting the weight down too fast, then when you try and stop it you might pull something. You are forcing the muscle to do more than it can safely do.

Second, you won't know how much weight you can actually handle. If you're swinging and using momentum on exercises, how do you know how many reps you actually did? What will you write in your book? "8 reps swung my body a little", or "10 reps swung a lot"?

Of course you are able to lift more weight if you swing or cheat on an exercise. Anyone can. But if you can't lift the weight with good form, you can't lift the weight. You are just not strong enough yet. Power lifters don't set world records with bent arms and legs. They have to do the exercise correctly or it doesn't count. It takes time to get strong, but follow the program with good form and focus on the task. It is safer and more motivating to have perfect form and see actual objective progress than to cheat and lift more weight with poor form. Just lower the weight. Your body will get stronger. It is literally impossible for it not too. Heavy weight will come, just stick to the plan.

Push as hard as you can and use your form as real time intel

I know when to stop an exercise when my form degrades. I don't stop the exercise because I reach a certain number of reps. Most beginners make this mistake. The program says "do 12" so they stop at 12. They could have done 15 but they stop at 12. It is called working out because you have to actually work the muscles. You need to tax the muscle or you won't see any gains.

Whatever your age, whatever your sex, do the exercise until you know you can't do another rep with good form. When you know that the next rep will have to be a cheat rep or you won't lift the weight, stop. Then write that number down in your notebook along with the weight. If you did 6 reps with a weight but were aiming for 8-12, then the weight was too heavy. If your form degraded and you stopped at 15 reps, then you know the weight was too light. Next set up the weight a little and see what you can do. This way we know without a doubt and without any subjective input from the wimpy voice what our body can do. This is how we track progress.

Ensure you know how to do the exercises correctly. And then do that exercise until your form doesn't allow you to do another rep. Use that number to set the weight. For examples on how to do each of the exercises in my program, go to my website, www.chrislehto.com. There are also thousands of videos on YouTube to explain the exercises if you need more direction.

Make sure you get full extension and full muscle flexion. Make sure your speed is consistent. The normal speed is 1 second contracting or pressing, and 2 seconds letting the weight down on the negative. We are always smooth and controlled and never jerk or release the weight too quickly. Don't let the weights slam on the racks. Controlled and smooth builds muscle. Controlled and smooth prevents injury.

Stop early if you feel pain, think long term

If you are feeling pain in your joints or ligaments at any time stop the exercise. The only times I have hurt myself lifting weights was when I kept lifting even though my body was telling me there was a problem. Stop immediately and assess. Do a different exercise or a different body part. Many people, including myself, have issues with shoulders and lower back. Those joints are the nexus for many different muscles and nerves. I am conservative when it comes to my shoulders or lower back.

My shoulder was complaining after doing close-grip bench press followed by bicep curls. Even though my body was telling me to stop, I continued and made the problem worse. I had to take the next two weeks off shoulders. I love those exercises, but for some reason my shoulders hurt afterwards.

Until your body adapts by getting stronger and more flexible you just have to work around the issue. There are hundreds, if not thousands, of different exercises out there to work each muscle group. All of them can be effective. Why do you think there are so many workout programs? What matters is that you max-perform your muscles with minimal stress on your joints and ligaments. You do that by pushing the muscles with good form and stopping as soon as there is an issue. Then just change the program to avoid the issue. After my shoulders gained strength and flexibility, I had no problems doing close-grip bench. I still have to be careful with barbell curls, but that day will come too. Your body will adapt. Just give it time. Start with a basic program and progress.

What if you start missing workouts or tracking data?

There is a saying in flying, "climb to cope." We use it on low-level flights. On low-level sorties we normally fly 500' above the ground at 500 mph. If you are very low to the ground and going really fast, it is difficult for missile systems to track you. There is too much clutter from the ground, trees, and mountains for the radar to get a clean return. And when they do get a clean return, you are going so fast that they can't actually track you until it's too late.

But low and fast has its downsides. The vast majority of air losses in the Vietnam War were from AAA. That is basically a large gun. Once the round leaves the chamber it is unguided, so if you are closer to the target (lower to the ground) it is easier to shoot you. If you are flying low to the ground, sometimes even a guy with a machine gun can get a lucky shot on a fighter. So the US decided to fly at higher altitudes and used stealth and electronic superiority to counteract the SAMs that could reach high altitudes.

The Brits and many other countries still go low, and they go much lower, because as a British Tornado pilot once told me, "When you're good at a game you stick with it…" It works great for them, the crazy bastards, but I have no doubt that they teach their pilots to "climb to cope" in an emergency or other problem. Basically, when you are that fast and that low, if you point your nose at the ground for a split second you will crash. I'm not exaggerating either. We review the time-to-die charts before each low-level phase. If you are 500 feet above the ground turning at 5 Gs and you overbank just 10 degrees, you will impact the ground in 5.7 seconds. In the air, 10 degrees is not even a noticeable amount.

No matter what is going on in the aircraft, you climb away from the ground before you start looking at something else. So we always get ourselves away from the biggest threat and buy some time to analyze what is going on and how to fix it. If we are having a hard time just keeping up with radio calls or our crosscheck is slow, we fly further away from the ground. We don't just quit, we continue the mission, but we pull it back a little bit.

If I notice my wingman is missing radio checks, or he is having a hard time staying in formation and targeting fighters or getting tally on ground targets, I will lower his task load. I will take over some of the responsibilities. It goes the same for me. If I start missing radio calls or my cross check is slow, I lower my task load and focus on what is important. I climb to cope. I make sure I'm hitting the most important tasks. We aviate first to make sure the plane doesn't hit the ground, then we navigate, and finally we communicate. We look outside and focus on the nearby rocks. Once our flight path is clear we can start to get situational awareness of our surroundings. Then we can start telling people about our position and situation.

If you notice you aren't keeping up with tracking your workouts or aren't going to the gym four times a week for some reason, pull back your task load. Focus on the main basic tasks of getting to the gym and tracking your workouts and body composition. If you have to shorten your workouts then shorten them, but hit your targets. Climb to cope, but finish the mission.

Remember, getting yourself in shape is the best investment you can make to live a longer and healthier life. Don't let the wimpy voice ruin your plans. Keep focused on the task. Use the tactics I highlighted to maximize results in less time in the gym. Maintain motivation by avoiding the SAM threats and use accurate and timely intel to constantly observe, orient, decide, and act. Keep it simple stupid! Avoid the threats and hit the targets. Don't make it more difficult than it needs to be, just make the task the priority and get the job done.

PART 3

NUTRITION

Chapter 10

Task 2: Start, Maintain, and Track a Food Plan

The second task is met when you have developed a system for food intake and have determined how much food is required to maintain your current weight. It should take approximately one month to determine your maintenance level of food intake.

Task 2: Start, Maintain and Track a Food Plan	
Targets:	*Primary* Use portion method or calorie tracker method to Write down what you eat Only consume fast-digesting carbs <1 hour after a workout *Secondary* Lose 0-2 lb. a week for men 0-1 lb. a week for women
Threats:	Hunger (enemy fighter) Unhealthy food temptations (SAMs) Low blood sugar levels (low fuel)
Tactics:	Burn fast fuel after a workout Eat more efficiently: replace fast-burning fuel with long-burning fuel Stay close to your maintenance level of energy Avoid and suppress unhealthy SAM threats Cheat to win with a cheat day once a week

Guns don't kill people, high velocity projectiles do

In air-to-air fighting it's not the enemy pilot that will kill you. It's not the enemy plane even. The actual instrument that kills is the weapon. If the enemy's gun doesn't fire or their missile fails to fuse then nothing will happen. You will live to fight another day. For this reason, we always fight the enemy weapons.

If we know they have long-range radar-guided missiles then we use tactics that will defeat radar. We turn sideways and descend. We make sure we have background clutter behind us and we dispense chaff that helps decoy the radar. If we know they have heat-seeking missiles then we try to stay out of their effective range of a few miles. But if we have to visually identify them we won't be able to stay out of range, so we lower our heat signature by pulling our throttle back. We also dispense hot burning flares that decoy heat-seeking missiles. If they have maneuvered into a gun solution then we have to jink by moving our plane out of the way of the bullets. It takes about a second for the bullets to fly a mile so you have one second to defeat the gunshot. There is no decoy for bullets.

On offense, we do the opposite. We use tactics to maneuver our aircraft into a position to use long-range radar missiles or shorter range heat-seeking missiles. If all else fails we get in close within a mile and use the cannon. You can't decoy the gun with flares or chaff and exploding rounds are dependable and effective.

A healthy diet is the truest weapon

Working out maneuvers your body into an offensive position. It gives your body the maneuvering room it needs to gain muscle or lose fat in the same way tactical fighter maneuvering allows you to get into a gun solution. Just getting into an offensive position at the enemy's six o'clock will not destroy the enemy plane. You need to put bullets through the plane. A healthy diet is the weapon that puts rounds on target.

My Pakistani fighter pilot buddy explained to me how he would work out for two hours a day. He would lift weights hard for an hour and then play competitive racquet ball for another hour. He never made any gains. He said he actually lost muscle. This is simply because he didn't eat enough food. He was in a position to make gains. His jet was sitting in the control zone, the enemy jet was right under his gun sight, but he couldn't close the deal. He was overworking to get in position. He was overflying the jet.

In this case, all that energy his muscles were using was coming from the muscles themselves. He was engaging the inefficient anaerobic processes, but he wasn't providing his body with the necessary ammunition to build muscle. You must provide the ammo to your body or you will not gain that much from working out. You will work your cardiovascular system and your muscles and ligaments will strengthen to a point. But you won't see real progress. Your strength gains will be minimal.

If my buddy had adjusted his diet too, he would have made amazing gains over that same period. Working out is required to get your body in a position to make gains, but the deal-closer is what you eat.

If a healthy diet is so important why not make it Task 1?

Working out maneuvers your body into a position to make faster and sustained gains. Your body will simply be stronger and more capable. You will see progress in the notebook within a few weeks, which is a good motivator. Once we have an established fitness regimen on autopilot, we can focus strictly on food. Again, we don't just take someone right out of college and start flying them in fighters. First they learn how to taxi, take-off, and land. Then they learn instruments and formation.

Working out is about taking action. You say you are going to do something difficult and then you get off your ass and actually do it. Everyone sees you going to work out and you get sweaty and feel good. You do it for a month and you force your wimpy voice to just sit in the back and keep its mouth shut. You are doing something active to make positive changes in your life. Completing the first task is a very important step because now we will focus on changing what you eat, and it is a lot less glamorous and more difficult. In Task 1, you learned how to correctly taxi, take-off, and land. You can make time for a fitness regimen: do it, and track your progress, so we can focus on the fighting.

Are you going to have a healthy and balanced diet right away? No, definitely not. Every new pilot is really terrible simply because they don't have the proper information. It takes time to learn all the intricacies of flying. No one in this world knows the ideal diet for you. If any program or person claims otherwise they are wrong.

The good news is that without a doubt, each day you can make positive changes that will add up over time. After a month, you will have a sustainable long-term diet in place. Diet might seem like the wrong word though. I could not find a word in the English language to describe food intake without the negative connotations of calorie restriction. But actually it's our cultural associations with "dieting" as a restrictive activity we do to lose weight that makes us perceive "a diet" as negative. So instead of "diet," I will use the word "food plan" to describe the types and amount of food that we should eat in our program to get our bodies into amazing shape.

We usually think of diets as restricting calories. But many times, including right now, I do not restrict my caloric intake at all. I am actually trying to eat more food energy than my body needs. I am not on a weight-loss plan, but I am following a basic food plan that will help me reach my current goal of adding muscle mass.

Chapter 11

Our 100-Year-Old Calorie System Is Incorrect

The last time I checked, there wasn't a fire burning-oven in my stomach. But that is precisely how we determine the caloric content of food. The basic assumptions about calories are wrong. Ridiculously, we still use the Atwater system which was developed over a hundred years ago. Seriously!? We can't figure out a solution to the obesity epidemic and yet we are still using a system we developed before airplanes.

And really the system is dumb. In order to determine the caloric content of a food we put a small amount of it in a container and burn it. The calorie assumptions you have used your entire life of 4 calories per gram for carbohydrates and protein, and 9 calories per gram for fat were found in this exact manner. It is extremely probable that these numbers are not correct for how our body actually uses the compounds.

Heat combustion, or fire, occurs when we combine fuel and an oxidant, usually oxygen, to create an energy releasing process. Your gas stove, for instance, works like this:

Fuel (propane) + oxygen → water + carbon dioxide + heat

In contrast, our body uses three completely different processes and the first two don't even use oxygen. For this reason they are called anaerobic processes. The third process does use oxygen, but at body temperature. The three systems our cells use are:

1. ATP-phosphocreatine system (provides the first 12 seconds of high power movement),
2. Glycolytic system (provides the second 13-50 seconds of moderate power movement),
3. Aerobic oxidative system (provides the final 51 seconds to hours of low power movement).

Here is where it gets interesting; the anaerobic processes are very fast metabolically, but extremely inefficient. The aerobic process is much slower but is 15 times more efficient. In the anaerobic processes one glucose molecule yields only two molecules of ATP, which is the actual fuel our muscles use, adenosine triphosphate. The aerobic oxidative system turns that exact same glucose molecule into 37 ATP molecules.

This is an important concept so let me summarize. The anaerobic high power processes make 2 ATPs and the aerobic process makes 37 ATPs from the same amount of chemical fuel. When that StairMaster machine displays the calories you've "burned," is it basing that number on the aerobic pathway or the two anaerobic pathways? Aerobic you say. Okay now how about when you do a set of 10 squats to failure, how many calories are you going to use? You don't know, you say? That is probably true because NO ONE KNOWS.

It gets better, because our bodies use all three systems at the same time. When you are on that StairMaster you are also using anaerobic processes. The burning sensation in your legs is most likely due to lactic acid buildup from the anaerobic process. I say most likely, because recent studies contradict this long-held assumption. We just don't know as much as we think we know about how the body works.

Our current caloric expenditure measurements are based solely on estimates of the aerobic pathway. But if my cells are using one of the anaerobic pathways then I use that same amount of glucose at 15 times the rate. This is not included in any of our assumptions about calories, because these are over a hundred years old. It should not be that hard to stay skinny in the modern world...unless the basic assumptions about our food and how our bodies actually use that food are wrong.

If anyone was really serious about fighting the obesity epidemic they would develop an accurate process for determining energy from food. If you are a scientist with the skills and motivation to try and find a better system, contact me at my website.

Yes if you light a gram of avocado on fire it will produce more energy than a gram of sugar. But that doesn't mean anything when we eat it. My stomach doesn't light the food on fire. When you eat sugar it is processed by little enzymes very quickly and the glucose enters your blood stream almost instantaneously. The glucose flows from the blood into the cells with the help of insulin released by the pancreas. Then your cells use the glucose by one of the three metabolic processes I just explained. If you don't use the energy right away then most likely it is stored in your body as fat.

On the other hand, the carbs, fat, and other nutrients, like fiber, in the avocado are digested more slowly over a longer period of time. Your pancreas doesn't release nearly as much insulin so the glucose is not processed quickly. There is no energy spike and since the food is absorbed more slowly, your body can use it over a longer period of time. It won't go straight to fat.

But according to our current system, the gram of avocado has over twice the calories of a gram of sugar and since it contains a lot of fat it will make you fat. From my own experience and understanding of biochemistry this is completely wrong.

If the system is wrong...find your own system

Ever wonder why there are so many different diets on the market? There are vegetarian, vegan, paleo, juice, south beach, north beach, and east beach diets. There are so many diets it would take forever to list them. I believe everyone really is different, so what works for you won't work for me. But another important factor is that the baseline assumptions are so wrong that everyone is just guessing. In the end, when we stop eating half the food we were eating, of course we will lose weight. But we will also crush our metabolism and hormone balance.

Fad diets are not sustainable in the long term. When you finish the diet, your body will put the fat right back on. I still believe it all depends on the amount of energy we give our bodies, but the way we are approaching it is just wrong. Our bodies are extremely adaptable. Our success on this planet is due in no small part to our amazing ability to eat literally everything else alive. I've been stationed in Korea and have traveled through Asia. I once saw a group of Korean children at a festival going crazy over a vendor's vat. I walked closer to see what candy they were eating and it was grilled silk worms. We can eat everything and there is a diet for everything.

The whole point of this task is to determine what works for the trillions of tiny living cells that make up your own body. Don't "diet," instead, arm yourself with a food plan optimized by and for you. The food plan that works for you will not necessarily work for me. Since the calorie numbers we are using are probably wrong if you track the type and amount of food you put into your own system and use the OODA loop process to learn the results then you will know without a doubt your own food plan. Our current "food science" is terrible, but through years of trial and error we have stumbled upon techniques that do work for most people. I believe the biggest problem is fast-burning carbohydrates consumed in a non-anabolic stage (after workout). This is why cutting these foods out of your food plan, unless you just worked out, is a primary target.

"Wow, You Look Great, How Did You Lose So Much Weight?"

I asked that question to a female acquaintance after not seeing her for several months. There was a lull in the conversation after she answered, "Oh I had giardia…"

Not eating is a very effective weight-loss technique. When we subtract a huge amount of food from our normal intake, such as the currently popular no-carb diets, yes, we will lose weight, but at a high cost. After millions of years on the savannah our ancestors' bodies developed techniques to survive. When food was plenty, their bodies saved the extra energy as fat. Just like a bear can survive a whole winter with minimal food, our ancestors were able to survive scarcity and famine thanks to stores of fat. But the problem is that the body does not give up fat easily. It will give up muscle as well. Yes, you can lose weight by not eating but you will also lose your hard-earned muscle.

Although we like to assume our body is like a car, burning calories and burning fat, our bodies are complex organic machines. From my experience, if you starve your body it will go into starvation mode. If you don't give it enough food it will start looking for resources inside the body. The body does not want to deplete its fat reserves, especially during a famine, so it will provide you with less energy and start using muscle and fat reserves. That is why we have no energy when we go on extremely low calorie/low carb diets. My cue that I am not eating enough food is getting light headed when I stand up.

Ever heard of the see-food diet? How about the no-food diet?

A remarkable experiment was published in the *British Medical Journal* in 1974. Somehow the researchers were able to track the weight loss—and specifically the protein loss from urinary nitrogen excretion—of 76 fasting patients. For an entire month, these 58 females and 18 males ate nothing. Nothing! And we complain about skipping a meal or two. I love this line in particular, "The therapeutic regimen consisted simply of no food."[9] My second favorite line in the study is "Patients were weighed daily after rising and emptying the bladder." The urine was analyzed for its nitrogen and potassium content.

The amount of nitrogen and potassium in the urine allowed the researchers to determine lean tissue degradation which is

---

[9] J. Runcie and T.E. Hilditch, "Energy Provision, Tissue Utilization, And Weight Loss In Prolonged Starvation," *British Medical Journal* 2 (1974): 352.

composed of protein and water. All the patients lost a lot of weight. It turns out that if you eat nothing for a month you will lose weight. But there was a significant difference between the first 14 days and the second 16 days. In the first two weeks of starvation the average weight loss was 8.3% of initial body weight for males and 7.4% for females. The average loss in the second half of the experiment was only 4.95% and 4.17% for males and females, respectively. The weight lost from initial body weight during the first 14 days was double the weight lost during the second 16-day period.

The researchers concluded that this large difference was because the lean tissue degradation was very high in the first couple weeks of starvation (based on urinary nitrogen levels) and then it tapered off when the body transitioned to using fat as the sole source (95% fat use to 5% lean tissue use). Until the starving body learns to use fat to fuel the nervous system it will use protein.

> [Protein's] comparatively large-scale catabolism in the initial period of fasting is due to a continuing dependence of the central nervous system on protein derived glucose as a metabolic substrate (Cahill et al, 1966). The subsequent switch of nervous tissue to direct utilization of the products of fat breakdown reduces body demand for glucose.[10]

So basically if you go into starvation mode, your body will use the glucose in your blood and then cannibalize the muscles for their glucose until the central nervous system can switch to using fat directly. Meanwhile, the fat loss of the patients was basically constant the whole time. This is why so much less weight was lost during the second half of the study. After the muscle catabolism, the patients' bodies learned to use fat as a primary source of energy.

It's as if a car could burn the seat upholstery for fuel. It would like to use the gas in the gas tank, but if it thinks there is no gas station for miles it will make use of other less critical things first.

---

[10] Runcie and Hilditch, "Energy Provision," 355.

You can still get to your destination with no upholstery but you will be sitting on metal benches. But if you run out of gas, you end up stuck on the side of the road. This is what it's like if there is no food around. Your body will use the muscles first and save the fat as a backup.

Remind your body there is a gas station around the corner

You need to coax the fat off your body. You want to skip the first 14 days and go direct to the second half of the study where lean tissue degradation is minimal and fat loss is still consistent. Starving may work for some people, but I believe for the majority of people a slight food energy deficit combined with whole body exercise is the most effective method.

You don't have to starve yourself to lose weight. Yes you will lose weight, but it will most likely be unlivable and you will also lose a lot of muscle. You just need to create a small enough energy deficit for your body to start using its fat reserves. The deficit should not be so large that your body starts protecting its fat reserves at the expense of muscle. If you are in an energy deficit for long enough you can teach your nervous system to use fat directly while still maintaining muscle. It's okay to be a little hungry, but if you are dying for food then you are doing it wrong.

My basic assumption is that the whole calorie-counting system is skewed. The grams are probably correct on the food labels but the calories and basic assumptions of what happens after we eat them are wrong. Protein has been shown time and time again to be critical for muscle growth and maintenance while fats and carbohydrates are our basic energy sources. You want a healthy supply of protein to build muscle and enough carbohydrates and fats to power your body during the day and during your workouts. If you can gently adjust your hormone levels to a reasonable level, you won't crave sugar and simple carbohydrates as much. You can actually train your body to use more fat.

There are many diets and techniques out there, but the food plan I recommend as a starting point is the one I have seen work successfully for myself and many people who have worked hard to get in shape. This balanced food plan has a rough breakdown of 35% carbohydrate, 35% protein, and 30% fat (by calorie). If you want to make it even simpler you can just call it the 1/3 food plan since you are eating a basic breakdown of 1/3 of each macronutrient. Once you track what you eat for a few weeks, you will see what works for you and can refine it using the OODA loop process.

The other primary target is to limit your consumption of fast-digesting carbohydrates to within 1 hour after a strenuous workout. Think of it as a reward for your hard work. As I will discuss later in this chapter, there is solid research indicating that within the anabolic window after a workout, fast-digesting carbs like sucrose are very beneficial to muscle repair and recovery. There is also very strong evidence that outside of this anabolic window fast-digesting carbs create fat.

This is a starting point because everyone's body chemistry is a little different. You have different bacteria in your gut than I do or the person next to you. Current science does not come close to understanding the intricacies of the digestive system. We still base much of our health information on what happens when you burn the food, not on how it is broken down and absorbed in the stomach, large intestine, and small intestine. For this reason I honestly cannot recommend a perfect food plan. Until we have testing to analyze what is actually in your gut to give us a breakdown, we won't know what will work the best, certainly per individual, except by trial and error and optimizing our food plan as we go. But I can give some general guidelines that have worked for me and that I have seen work for others.

Don't change everything at once…

Most people start a diet way too aggressively. They are motivated at the beginning and try to change all their eating habits at once. It takes a ton of willpower to change all our habits at once. Changing more than a few things at once usually results in failing at all of them. That is why this is Task 2. After we get moving and have a program firmly in place we can start to work on our eating habits.

Your eating habits have been formed over decades. Trying to change them in a week or even a month is a recipe for failure. In fighter training we don't just toss a new student into full air-to-air or air-to-ground combat. We first teach them 1v1 dogfighting. Once they have proven they can do it, we move on to 2v1 air combat maneuvering. When they have learned that then they move on to tactical intercepts. After tactical intercepts, finally we get to full-on air-to-air combat maneuvering. Each phase is 3-4 flights and normally, students don't pass them all.

You should approach your food plan the same way. Think long term. You cannot change all the bad things you eat in a month and manage to stick with the plan. This is why so many people fail. They go too hard and fast at the beginning only to find the effort requires too much willpower. I don't have any problem turning down food 95% of the time. No matter what the food is. The other 5% of the time I either use willpower to turn it down or I just eat it. Just like brushing my teeth it has become a habit. So I plan ahead to avoid the threats.

If I can't avoid the threats or if a pop-up threat arises, I suppress it. If that doesn't work I just eat the food. We still have to enjoy life and I enjoy food. There are only a few foods in this world I don't enjoy. It's difficult for me to live in Italy during mushroom season. But I don't have to eat ice cream every day. If I go off my plan, I enjoy what I eat and move on. I don't give up on the plan just because I ate something not on it. We don't just quit, we stay on target. Motivation will come and go. Just like the stock market we will have ups and downs. Remember if you continue on an upward trajectory, you can't fail in the long run.

The bottom line is that it takes years to make a combat-ready pilot. We go phase by phase, ensuring the student passes each phase of the training. You won't be able to completely overhaul your diet in a month without exerting a ridiculous amount of willpower. It can be done, but your chance of success is much lower. If you take the long view though, make small positive changes in your food plan and allow your body to adapt to those changes, you increase your chance of success exponentially.

It is not you that craves the sugary drinks and foods. It is your body, with the wimpy voice as its messenger. If you slowly change your food plan and ensure you have passed each phase, you will end up with a full-on air-to-air combat-ready food plan in a few months. The best part is you won't even be hungry or really miss the food and you still get to eat the food you love. I literally eat whatever I want. I just set limits on when I eat it and how much I eat. On cheat days I don't even limit it at all.

Don't over think it, just hit the primary and secondary targets

In this task your first primary target is to track a basic food plan for a month. I'll explain two methods to track your food plan later in this section. Your second primary target is to make a few changes to your current diet that will get you the biggest bang for your buck. Avoid high-glycemic carbs such as sugary drinks, desserts, or processed foods unless you've just worked out. Don't worry—you can eat all that terrible stuff on your cheat day.

Your secondary target is to make sure you don't overdo your food plan. Each week when you weigh yourself try to hit 0-1 pound weight loss per week for men and 0-.5 pound weight loss per week for women. You have hit your primary and secondary targets if you successfully track what you eat for a month and avoid sugary foods and drinks, unless you've just worked out, without increasing your weight. The key is to hit the primary targets.

Primary for a reason

The point of this task is to make a habit of knowing and tracking what you eat and when you eat it. By slowly making healthy modifications to your food intake you can make lasting changes that promote true change in your life. If you just stumble through a program and lose a few pounds, without a doubt you will put that weight back on sooner rather than later.

We are creatures of habit. I have confidence that I will perform under combat stress because the actions are so ingrained in me that I won't have to think about it. I will just do it. I don't drink sugary drinks unless I worked out in the previous hour. I don't have to think about it. I simply don't do it. This is what we want from your eating habits. You won't have any problem sticking to a certain food plan because it is just what you eat. It is who you are.

The secondary targets are to make sure you don't go crazy with your food plan. Once you start tracking what you eat I guarantee you will eat healthier. The problem is that most people eat too healthy and too little. When you start avoiding sugary drinks and foods you will see how much sugary food you actually eat. It is most likely a lot.

You don't want to put your body into starvation mode and you don't want to make the food plan unlivable. By just tracking what you eat and being cognizant of what and how much food you are putting in your body, you will start to change your habits.

Your target is to maintain your weight or decrease it by no more than 1 lb. per week for men or 0.5 lb. per week for women. The maximum amount of weight you want to lose is 2 lb. per week for men and 1 lb. per week for women. Any more weight loss than that and I believe most people go into starvation mode and lose too much muscle. Everyone is different though, so if you still have energy and your motivation is high then you can go to the maximum numbers, but I believe it is unnecessary.

If you did the math on the maximum weight loss numbers, it is going to take you ten weeks to lose 20 lb. of fat if you are a man or 10 lb. of fat if you are a woman. Deal with it. That is how long it takes to change your body and your habits. Is it really that long anyway?

People think short term. We want to make a life change but want it to happen in one month. It doesn't work that way. Don't listen to the wimpy voice. No matter what anyone says on TV or anywhere else, for the vast majority of the population 2 lb. a week is how long it takes.

The good part is in this program you will be losing mostly fat. If you lose more than 2 lb. (men) or 1 lb. (women) a week then you are most likely also losing muscle. Fat is energy-dense and it takes an energy deficit along with the correct hormones to coax the fat cells to give up their energy. That is the maximum most people can do. Hit these targets over a long enough period of time and you will get fit, with the body to match. It is math. If your food plan is livable and you are making it a priority then you can't fail.

Chapter 12

Nutrition Threats

Hunger Is the Biggest Threat

There are a lot of threats when dealing with a food plan but the biggest threat we have to deal with is hunger. Hunger is the enemy air-to-air fighter. We all have a finite amount of willpower and I don't know about you but I have a hard time constantly turning down unhealthy food if I am hungry. When I am not hungry I have no problem turning down ice cream or fast-food. But as soon as I am hungry it is a whole different ballgame. My ability to hold back the wimpy voice is diminished. I think, "maybe if I just eat a little bit then I won't be as hungry anymore and that will be enough." After a few bites I am actually hungrier so I keep eating.

When we are hungry food just tastes better doesn't it? I starved out in the woods for a week during survival training and the whole time we talked about food. Every single conversation around the campfire, while hiking, or trying to evade simulated bad guys went back to different types of food. I had a big football player in my group of ten cadets. He was a running back and he was really hungry, all the time. He happily ate the extra rabbit lung I couldn't chew down. All he ever talked about was food. I remember him just staring into the fire talking about cheeseburgers. The first day back I had a greasy hamburger with French fries and it was one of the best meals I've ever had. My stomach hurt like crazy and I felt terrible after but it was amazing. I like a hamburger as much as the next guy but this meal was a level above.

Hunger is why most people say "screw it" and blow their diets. The problem is most people just hit hunger head-on. They think that skinny, well-trained people just fight through the hunger pains and are able to just not eat the unhealthy foods. This is not true. They just know how to avoid hunger pains in the first place.

In one very large air-to-air exercise I flew as the Red-Air simulated enemy forces. We purposely overtasked the Blue Defensive Counter-Air defense fighters. There were simply too many Red-Air fighters for the good guy pilots to deal with. They didn't have enough missiles. After many failed exercise days the good guys came up with a new plan that finally allowed them to win. It was an ingenious tactic you may have heard of. They ran away.

For the first couple of weeks the good guys kept beating their heads against the problem head-on. But, outgunned and outmanned, they simply couldn't win using normal offensive tactics. The day the Blue forces figured out the tactic, they were losing ground to the Red-Air like all the other days. But then, by accident, at the same exact time across the airspace, the Blue fighters flew backwards away from the threat. We watched it in the debriefing on the massive screen. Maybe they were just tired of getting shot like the other days but on the screen it looked like watching a football game and all the defending players just turned around and ran towards their own goal.

Then something happened, as the Red forces were chasing the Blue fighters they started to turn around. The Red forces were running out of gas. When only a few Red-Air remained the Blue-Air turned around and quickly swept the entire airspace clean. As the Red forces we were all happy for the Blue-Air. It doesn't sound like a good tactical plan on paper and not something you would brag about to your fighter buddies in the bar, but running away had worked.

But this isn't the mentality of a fighter pilot you say! Fighter pilots never run away right? Wrong. Of course we run away...if that is what it takes to win. We do whatever it takes to win. No one said we couldn't turn cold for a few minutes. Admittedly, it is not the toughest tactic in the world but in the right situation it works. Hunger is the same threat. It is always there and sometimes there are just too many enemy fighters. Sometimes you find yourself at a party with your favorite foods surrounding you, you are hungry, and you just finished a very tough week. You will try to shoot your way out and hit the enemy threats head-on. "I will just power through it." Or so we think.

Most people think they will just suffer through the diet with willpower. In fact, when you even think the word "diet," I bet "suffer" and "willpower" come to mind too. You don't have to suffer and you don't have to constantly fight against hunger to be successful. But you do have to cheat and plan ahead. Sometimes you have to just run away. Willpower can work but it is extremely difficult and I believe it's the reason most people fail. If we are open to different ideas and think long term our chance of success is much higher.

Unhealthy food temptations

After we deal with the enemy fighters we have to deal with the surface-to-air missile (SAM) systems. If we know where the SAM is then the best way to deal with it is to just avoid it. If you can't turn down a Krispy Kreme doughnut, or whatever your poison, because they are amazingly delicious, then the easiest plan is to just not be around Krispy Kreme doughnuts. Be outside the Krispy Kreme doughnut's maximum effective range. For a modern SAM system that number can be anywhere from 10-100 miles. Doughnuts are much smaller, but I would still say you need to be outside smelling and sight range.

If you stop by a fast-food restaurant and eat a horrible breakfast on your way to work every day just avoid the SAM by not stopping in its range ring. Take a different route to work. You can pass through the threat range ring quickly but as soon as you sit there and loiter you are giving the enemy more time to find and target you.

Every minute you stay inside a food's threat ring is another minute you have to use willpower to counter it. We don't want to use our willpower. We want to preserve it for pop-up threats. But if we have to stay inside a threat ring for an extended period of time we must suppress it. The easiest way to suppress hunger pains is to not be hungry. Eat something healthy instead of the junk food. Like dealing with real SAM systems, suppressing hunger pains requires advance planning. It's not as difficult as it sounds but it's the primary reason I recommend supplements as a tactic. Supplements allow us to quickly and easily replace an unhealthy food for a healthier one by not being hungry inside a threat ring. If you are not hungry then you can sit inside a threat ring untargeted. It can be any healthy food actually, but supplements are easier to use for many of us. In the end, you should use whatever works for you.

Low blood sugar levels: Maximize range

Before every fighter mission we meticulously plan our fuel use. If a plane runs out of fuel the options are pretty limited. You can't just pull over and stop. You can glide to an airfield but you have to be within approximately 20 miles to glide to it. I also imagine it is not a pleasant experience for the pilot. Luckily, I haven't had to do it.

On every flight, starting from the first mission in pilot training, fuel is always in the back of our minds. Now it is a habit. I am constantly checking my fuel burn and fuel remaining. I do it automatically. In the mission planning, we agree to tactics, routes, and time over target based on our available fuel. If we need more then we have to plan for aerial refueling.

Your blood glucose levels should be thought of as your fuel. As soon as your body runs out of fuel it is going to initiate hunger pains and you will be gliding to the nearest fast-food restaurant. You will not be able to do anything productive and at that point you could actually be a hindrance to the mission.

When my body runs out of gas I get grumpy, difficult to deal with, and I start making bad decisions. I will eat whatever is in arms reach, the more sugary and unhealthy the better. We crave sugar or fast-processing food because this type of food enters our blood stream immediately. My body knows this. If there is a salad or a candy bar to choose from, the candy bar looks ten times more tempting. This is the situation we want to avoid. It is not good for anyone, especially our friends and family.

In order to not run out of gas we need to provide our body with long-range foods. I would say slow-burning foods, but they aren't actually burned, are they? This means if you just eat cereal for breakfast, I bet you are grumpy and pretty hungry by around 10:30. You might crave some bad snacks around that time also. But if you eat eggs, bacon, vegetables, and nuts for breakfast I bet you aren't hungry until lunch time.

Chapter 13

Tactics to Avoid Nutrition Threats and Hit Targets

So the three main threats we are concerned with for our food plan are the ever present enemy fighters of hunger, the ground-located surface-to-air missile (SAMs) threat of unhealthy food, and the body fuel glucose levels. Now we need to develop the tactical techniques and procedures we are going to use to hit the targets and avoid the threats.

Let's start with our first primary target, track a basic food plan for 1 month. Tracking a food plan is similar to fuel mission planning. In fuel mission planning, until you gain some experience, or in unusual situations, the best game plan is to use a computer. For fighter planning we use a dedicated mission planning program. We meticulously enter all our flight conditions including altitudes, airspeeds, and winds based on what bombs, missiles, and other pods we are carrying on the jet. It takes a long time to navigate through the US contractor-produced software. Like all computer programs it can be a pain to use, so we task the newest, youngest pilot to the software.

The computer software may be a pain to use, but in the end we know very accurately how far we will fly and if we will make it to our destination. This is the most accurate and dependable way to gauge fuel considerations or to gauge caloric intake. If your food plan is very consistent from day-to-day, you only have to calculate once or twice. Then you can just record the "same as yesterday". It really isn't as difficult as it sounds. After 13 years of flying fighters I can just measure the distances we will fly on a map and make a rough-guess estimate of our fuel requirements. It is not as accurate as a computer, but it lets me know if I need to use the computer.

The best technique I have seen was accomplished by the Italians at the European Tactical Leadership Program. As mission commander I asked the Italians if they could make it to the long-range target. The flight lead pulled a long string out of his flight suit. He expertly placed the string on the map along their route of flight and said "Yes, no problem". He also had a way with words. "You Americans are good at war. We Italians are good at air shows…"

After you have tracked your food plan for a month you will be able to just pull out the string and make rough-guess estimates of how much energy you are consuming. I still recommend you write down what you are eating for each meal, but your estimates of energy will always be much more accurate if you have been meticulously tracking your food plan up to that point.

Since the calories are skewed, by writing down what you are actually eating you can make changes to your food plan to reach your targets. In the end, do what you will continue to do for the long haul. I use the smartphone app MyFitnessPal. It is easy to use and helps me keep track of all my food. At the end of the day I just see how many calories and macronutrients are left and I drink a protein shake to cover the difference.

Eat more efficiently

The first question people normally ask me about flying fighters is "how fast do you go?" The answer is it depends. If we are using the afterburner and literally pouring jet fuel into the nozzle and lighting it on fire, then we can go up to twice the speed of sound (approximately 1200 mph at altitude). It's called an afterburner because the fuel is sprayed into the exhaust gases in the nozzle and lit on fire after the gas is compressed and burned inside the engine core. It's like pouring gas into the exhaust pipe of your car and lighting it on fire. We can go really fast but it is horribly inefficient. After about 6-9 minutes in afterburner we will use all of our fuel.

However when we are dogfighting, afterburner is required because it provides up to 50% more thrust. That is a big difference in a fighter. A fighter with an afterburner will own a non-afterburner fighter. There is no use saving gas if you are dead, so we use the afterburner to maneuver our aircraft into an offensive position. If we are doing long-range fighting we don't normally use afterburner unless we are escaping to avoid being inside a missile employment zone. As we get further away from the enemy there is less to gain by just lighting our gas on fire. We conserve energy so we have it when we need it. In day-to-day admin flying we fly the same speed as an airliner and never use afterburner. We get the most efficient use of our fuel.

Burn fast fuel after a workout

Fast-digesting carbohydrates such as liquid sugars are the afterburner for your body. Like afterburner they provide a huge benefit when your body can use the fast energy but come at a cost when your body can't use the energy. Immediately following a workout is a perfect time to eat high-glycemic carbs because our body needs the high dose of energy to fuel muscle repair and to restore glycogen and ATP. Unfortunately if we eat the fast-digesting carbs at other times -when our body can't use the energy, we will gain fat.

In the outstanding book *Nutrient Timing*, authors John Ivy Ph.D. and Robert Portman Ph.D. explain through the use of many clinical studies how fast-digesting carbohydrates combined with a smaller amount of protein increases muscle gains, increases fat loss, and limits soreness when taken immediately following workouts. The best ratio found in clinical trials at the University of Texas in Austin and corroborated by further studies at Vanderbilt University was 3 grams of high-glycemic carbs such as sucrose, maltodextrine, and dextrose to 1 gram of protein. The best time was within 1 hour after working out with diminishing results up to 4 hours after workout. The actual grams are 40-50 g carbs and 13-15 g whey protein (three to one carbs to protein ratio).

The authors recommend whey protein because it has several advantages. To name a few, it is fast acting, has all nine amino acids, and has a higher concentration of branched-chain amino acids (BCAAs) than any other protein source. One disadvantage is that it contains lactose. The authors also recommend that 1-2 g of leucine, 1-2 g glutamine, 60-120 mg of vitamin E, and 80-400 IU of vitamin C should be added to the post-workout drink.

If you have any misgivings or questions concerning the science or logic behind this post-workout drink then you should definitely read *Nutrient Timing*. Its arguments are backed by sound reasoning and solid science.

You can drink fruit juice, eat ice cream, or whatever you want as long as it has simple sugars. Not only do you get to eat and drink the things you normally shouldn't, but it also benefits you. Ivy and Portman found that those people who drank simple sugars after resistance training gained more muscle and lost more fat than those athletes that drank only water or protein drinks. The simple sugars were found to be more important than protein, but the most effective combination was simple sugars mixed with a little bit of protein (3 g sugars/1 g protein).

This is an example of how we can eat what we want and still stay within our food plan. We just have to change when we eat the foods that might otherwise be unhealthy. Move the sugary foods to within 60 minutes after your workout and combine a little bit of protein, and you are actually increasing your gains. The high-glycemic carbs cause the pancreas to release more insulin. The higher levels of insulin make it easier for proteins to be shuttled into the muscle cells. The muscles replenish glycogen stores and repair themselves faster. The end result is more muscle and strength gains, more fat loss, and less soreness and injuries.

I use supplements for this post-workout drink because it is convenient, effective, and tastes good. If you don't want to use supplements then just create your own post-workout drink that contains the same nutrients. Ivy and Portman recommend a liquid drink because it metabolizes faster than solid food.

Fly at maximum range airspeed if you aren't fighting

In normal day-to-day operations fast-digesting carbohydrates, like afterburner, just use fuel too quickly and are not necessary. Try a simple experiment. One day eat just cereal for breakfast and note how your morning goes and how hungry you are at lunchtime. The next day eat the caloric content of your cereal in the form of eggs and cheese. Now note the difference in how much energy you have and how hungry you are by lunchtime. Because the eggs and cheese have more fat and protein in them, you will be less hungry.

If you are going to work out within a half hour or so, your body will use the fast-digesting carbs very effectively during the workout. Working out is like dogfighting, our bodies will use the excess energy to tear and repair muscles. In that case, go ahead and eat the fast-digesting carbs prior to your workout. That is why we work out, so we can gain the strength benefits and make our food plan much easier to maintain.

But if you are not going to work out immediately or didn't just work out, stay away from the fast-digesting carbohydrates and especially liquid carbohydrates. Liquid carbohydrates such as fruit juices metabolize extremely quickly and will spike your insulin levels. Spiked insulin levels help greatly after a strength training workout but will promote fat gain any other time.

Replace fast-burning fuel with long-burning fuel

Our first tactic to combat hunger is to get more protein and fat into our food plan at the expense of fast-digesting carbohydrates. Examples of fast-digesting carbs are any sugar, white bread, pastries, crackers, and potato chips. Basically, if you throw it in a pond for the ducks how long does it stay whole? A piece of white bread dissolves pretty quickly. If you throw in wholegrain bread it takes quite a bit longer. If you toss a potato or a bean in it lasts for many hours. We want proteins to replace the fast-digesting carbohydrates and especially any liquid carbs. Most people get enough fats in their normal diet so don't cut those out, just like carbohydrates, fats are part of a healthy balanced diet. The real problem is sugar (which is in everything in America).

According to the chairman of the department of nutrition at the Harvard School of Public Health, "if Americans could eliminate sugary beverages, potatoes, white bread, pasta, white rice and sugary snacks, we would wipe out almost all the problems we have with weight and diabetes and other metabolic diseases" ("A Reversal on Carbs," *Los Angeles Times*, December 20, 2010). I don't think this is entirely correct. Vegetables such as potatoes and rice quench hunger and have other vitamins and nutrients. They need not be completely avoided like sugary drinks.

I believe diets such as the Atkins diet work because when you remove the fast-digesting carbohydrates you make your body use fat as an energy source. But those types of extreme diets are very difficult to live with and are not effective in the long term.

In a long-term follow up to the starvation therapy treatment, 1 in 4 of the patients was successful.[11] If that seems high to you, remember that these people were motivated enough to literally starve for an entire month. The fact that only 25% of the participants in the 30-day starvation study saw long-term success should be evidence that starving is not a viable long-term diet (although it apparently can be effective for 25% of those people crazy enough to try it).

As further evidence that the short term fad diets don't work, when Atkins died he weighed 258 lb., so chances are high he was unable to follow his own diet in the long term ("Just What Killed the Diet Doctor, And What Keeps the Issue Alive?" *New York*

---

[11] J.A. Innes et al., "Long-term Follow-up of Therapeutic Starvation," *British Medical Journal* 2 (1974):356-59

Times, February 11, 2004). Carbs are part of a healthy balanced diet and will help your body build strength and endurance. Removing a whole food group from your food plan is just a bad idea. You want a food plan that is healthy, doable, and still allows you to enjoy food. If you just keep your carbs to approximately 1/3 of your intake you will develop a more efficient metabolism but you will still get to enjoy delicious carbohydrates and give your body ammo to gain strength.

A second, ancillary—but very important—reason for including carbohydrates in our food plan is that they are delicious. I love carbohydrates. If I never ate carbs again my quality of life would be lower. I went without carbs for several months and I had no energy, my strength decreased, and I was lightheaded when I stood up. It was horrible.

How to choose long-range carbs

Not all carbohydrates are created equal. They do not all elicit the same response in the body. For the one-third of your food plan consisting of carbohydrates you should choose long-range carbohydrates. But how do you know which foods are long range? I have been referencing the glycemic index, but is that really the best way to choose a food? The glycemic index is based on the amount of blood sugar measured in a person's blood after eating a particular food. The index is based off a 100-point scale for white bread. When you eat a serving of white bread your blood sugar rises a certain amount and nutritionists call that 100. It is the gauge.

High-glycemic carbohydrates, or high GI carbs, have a high score relative to white bread's score. There are two major problems with the glycemic index. First it can only be used for carbohydrates, so you can't compare even "healthy" low glycemic carbohydrates to other foods such as protein and fat. If you measure the body's insulin response to the food you can compare proteins, fats, and carbohydrates. It is called the insulin index. The second major problem with the glycemic index is that the body doesn't react to foods in proportion with their glycemic index.

For instance, according to a 1997 study of the food insulin index, the only one I could find, jelly beans and crackers both scored 118. They cause higher blood sugar content than white bread at 100.[12] But the jelly beans spiked insulin higher than any other food in the study, up to 160. On the other hand, the crackers caused insulin levels to increase about half as much, to 87. Even though these jelly beans and crackers have the same glycemic index score, your body produces twice as much insulin when you eat jelly beans. Our tools for measuring food are not accurate.

Although I would not consider either food healthy, if you have to pick between jelly beans or crackers, pick the crackers (unless you just worked out and want to spike your insulin). This should make sense right? Jelly beans are straight sugar. I can feel my blood sugar spike after I eat jelly beans. Yet if we blindly follow the glycemic index we will have a hard time nailing down a food plan that works for us. The crackers actually raise insulin levels less than white bread but, according to their glycemic index, they cause a higher blood glucose level.

We do not fully understand the complex biochemical reactions inside the body. I believe insulin response is a better indicator of a food's impact on the body than glycemic index, but, at the time of writing, there is not a plethora of scientific information on the subject. The results of this study compared several common foods, and can be found here http://bit.ly/1V7Df8S. The most accurate way to learn what each food actually does to your particular biochemical system is to track what you eat and apply the OODA loop process. At the beginning I recommend you follow the few simple rules outlined in this book and then refine as you go.

---

[12] Susanne Holt et al., "An insulin index of foods: the insulin demand generated by 1000-kJ portions of common foods," *American Journal of Clinical Nutrition* 66, no. 5 (2009): 1264-76.

Start slow and don't change everything at once

In order to make the food plan livable, we want to maintain a small energy deficit over a long period of time. If you are already skinny then eat to maintain or even gain weight. We will teach your body to become more efficient by slowly and systematically replacing the fast-digesting foods with slow-digesting foods. Like the starvation patients learned firsthand, the body can use fat—it just has to be coaxed into doing it.

If we can remove the fast-digesting foods and remain energy neutral for an extended period of time our internal chemical engine will start to use fat as a primary energy source. Otherwise your body will rely on the constant supply of liquid sugar thrown right into the blood stream like an afterburner. Once that blood sugar is depleted in order to keep your metabolism going you have to throw more fuel on the fire and eat more fast-digesting foods. This is why we get an energy spike and then a bust with sugars. It's why kids go crazy after eating sugar and then crash and want more sugar. But just like dog fighting, when we need the energy we use the afterburner. After a tough workout is the perfect time to use energy inefficiently because it will benefit us and allow us to reach our goals faster.

At any other time besides within 60 minutes after a workout, avoid any fast-digesting carbohydrates that will spike your insulin. Avoid any sugar or highly processed breads like French bread, pretzels, doughnuts, croissants, most simple sugary cereals, and white bread. These foods can be hard to substitute, but vegetables and nuts are the healthiest replacements. Fruit is also a healthy replacement option, but bananas and grapes spike insulin the same amount as cake. Definitely don't drink any fruit juices. If you have to splurge, popcorn and potato chips have an insulin index score of 54 and 61 respectively, equivalent to brown rice.

Other common high insulin response carbohydrates are potatoes and white rice. In their place, eat white or brown pasta. Brown whole meal pasta was the best carbohydrate option in the study, with a surprisingly low insulin response of 40. It also had a lot of protein. Grain bread is also a good option at 56. I have personally had success with couscous and quinoa. Although it is controversial, potatoes and rice are whole food options that I believe can still have a place in a balanced food plan.

Start buying healthier options at the grocery store

Don't make it more complicated than it needs to be. Instead of buying processed food and sugary drinks at the grocery store, just buy the foods I highlighted above. Don't buy fruit juice, buy the fruit. Don't buy crackers, buy nuts. Instead of buying bread buy a supposedly low glycemic replacement. Instead of Hamburger Helper, buy steak and wholegrain brown pasta.

We also want to increase our protein intake and keep our fat intake around the same. Each macronutrient should make up about 1/3 of our total energy intake. Since it's all we have, estimate this energy intake with the misguided Atwater calorie system. You won't make good decisions in the grocery store when you are hungry, so make a list at home when you are not hungry. Once you start tracking what you actually eat you will quickly learn what the problem foods are.

Stay close to your maintenance level of energy

The second tactic we will use to battle ever present hunger is to not be in a crazy energy deficit. In order to lose weight, we have to eat slightly less usable energy than our body needs. There is a certain amount of energy that your body uses throughout the day. All the energy you use to move your muscles, power your brain, repair tissue damage, and countless other physiological processes is called your daily energy requirement. Go above this amount and you will be in an energy surplus, go below this amount and you will be in an energy deficit. If you are in an energy surplus you are going to gain weight. In a deficit you will lose weight. If you are working out and in a moderate energy deficit you should lose mostly fat. If you aren't working out and you are in a deficit you will lose both muscle and fat.

Most diets that I have seen use large energy deficits as their main tool. Take the Atkins diet for example. If you suddenly stop your carbohydrate intake, based on the average American diet, you will lose 55% of your daily calories. That can be over 1000 calories for a 160-pound man. Sure, you can replace the carbohydrates with hamburgers without the bun but you'll have to eat a lot of hamburgers without the bun to make up 1000 calories. Also those calories are not being counted very accurately to begin with. There is a real possibility that those carbohydrates make up an even larger portion of what your body is actually using as energy.

With an energy deficit as extreme as that, your body will go into starvation mode. Like my Pakistani buddy learned, you will have low energy and still not lose the fat you are trying to lose because your body will conserve its energy reserves. During the starvation therapy study, the first two weeks of starvation resulted in a high percentage of protein degradation.

You will also be very hungry as your body keeps sending strong signals to your brain to eat. If you can keep your caloric deficit to less than 500 calories as an initial starting point, you will be able to slowly teach your body to effectively use fat as an energy source. You will also be able to control your insulin without so many carbohydrates spiking your hormone levels. When your body does need fast-digesting carbohydrates to replenish glycogen and repair muscles, provide it shortly after workout. In this manner, you can limit protein degradation while losing fat.

Choose the nerd or cave person way

I recommend two techniques to implement our food plan. There is the math way and the caveman picture way. I believe both work, so pick one and try it out. You won't know what works for you until you try it. Also, keep in mind that the calorie numbers we are using are broad-based estimates based on a flawed system. Although our current calorie models are inaccurate, until a better system is developed they do give us a starting point.

If you enjoy using a smart phone to look up your food and share with your friends, go the math route initially. If you feel overwhelmed at the prospect of tracking everything in a smart phone then use the caveman picture way.

Since secretly most fighter pilots are nerds, I will explain the math technique first. We need to find the number of calories that will keep us close to our maintenance levels of calories. We are neither in a deficit nor a surplus. If we stay at the same weight but are working out consistently then we are losing fat and gaining muscle. Maybe slowly but that is what is happening as long as we are seeing progress in our workouts. This is what we want from a basic food plan. We want to maintain or be in a slight energy deficit.

Once we determine our maintenance level of calories and know our basic food plan then we can start tweaking the plan to build muscle faster or lose fat faster depending on our goals. For the first month determine your maintenance level of food intake by tracking what you eat and how much weight you gain or lose. This is the goal of our primary target.

How do we determine our maintenance level of food energy? What is the number of each macronutrient that is required to maintain our current weight? I like to have a simple game plan going out the door and then reassess in the air. Observe, orient, decide, and act. Let's use the KISS principle and start with some general rules of thumb. Take your body weight in pounds and multiply by 12. This is a rough estimate of your daily total caloric requirement. It includes working out 3-4 times a week.

Your weight in pounds equals your protein and carbohydrate requirements in grams. If you weigh 200 lb. you need to eat 200 grams of protein and 200 grams of carbohydrates a day. Now since fats are 9 calories per gram, divide your weight by 2 (instead of 4) and subtract 10% of that number. So if you weigh 200 lb. divide by 2 and subtract 10 (10% of 100) to get 90 grams of fat.

This leaves us with 200 grams of protein, 200 grams of carbs, and 90 grams of fats.

This is your target amount of macronutrients. If you eat that amount every day, you will hit your food goals for the day. If you do that consistently and compare it to your weekly weight and waist measurements you will know at the end of each week how you are doing. If the waist measurement is not decreasing or your weight is increasing too fast then the next week lower the carb amount by 10%.

Each week observe how your body is reacting. If you are on your progress line (either maintaining or losing no more than 2lb for men/1lb for women per week) then decide to stay the course and act by continuing your current food plan. If you observe you are gaining weight and your waist measurement is increasing, then decide to lower the carbs and act on the new food plan by buying different foods at the grocery store and so on. Lower the carbs twice and then start lowering the fats. The protein should be lowered last.

This is a basic muscle-building food plan. I didn't make it up. This type of food plan in differing ratios has worked for thousands of people over the last decade. A recent large-scale study called the Diet, Obesity and Genes (DioGenes) European multicenter trial investigated weight control in 932 obese families, specifically the "importance of a slight increase in dietary protein content, reduction in carbohydrate, and the importance of choosing low (LGI) vs high (HGI) carbohydrates".[13] Even after a year, the combination was "additive on weight loss and maintenance, and [was] successful in preventing weight regain and reducing drop-out rate".[14] This food plan will most likely work right off the bat.

And no, protein is not going to hurt your kidneys or liver or whatever other myths are out there. Fat is not bad for you either. Apart from the many studies over the past 20 years showing the

---

[13] A. Astrup, A. Raben and N. Geiker, "The role of higher protein diets in weight control and obesity-related comorbidities," International Journal of Obesity 39, no. 5 (2015): 721.

[14] A. Astrup, A. Raben and N. Geiker, "The role of higher protein diets,"721.

safety and benefits of protein powder, our ancestors lived on the plains of Africa eating wildebeest protein and fat by the kilo. I assure you that unless you have serious dietary restrictions one-third of your food plan can come from protein and another third from fat with no ill side effects. This is just a going-in game plan. If you are turned off by having to track all your calories in a calorie tracker then just use the caveman picture method.

The caveman picture method is otherwise formally called the portion method. All you do is hold your fist above your dinner plate. This is basically one-third of the plate. If you want to maintain or gain weight you eat one fist (portion) of protein, one fist of carbs, and one fist of vegetables.

If you are trying to lose weight then instead of the carbs you eat another portion of vegetables. Before and after your workouts you still eat carbs for the reasons I outline in Task 1, but eat veggies instead of carbs during the other meals, especially at night. You should also try to eat five or six smaller meals during the day separated by three hours or so. You should never feel overly full or have a food hangover. The two or three shakes you have throughout the day count as meals. The macronutrient content (carb, fat, protein) of your shakes should be similar in makeup to your meals.

You still need to write down what you eat each meal in your notebook for the portion tracking method, but otherwise that is all there is to it. On paper it looks easier than the calorie tracker to execute but I have found I like the calorie tracker method better. Both can be effective. Try one of the techniques and see how you like it. If that doesn't work try the other technique or a different technique entirely, but make sure you hit the primary targets. Track your food plan for a month and avoid sugar unless within 60 minutes after a workout.

Do whatever it takes to hit the primary targets. The secondary target is to maintain or slightly lower your weight. It is secondary to the primary targets. If you are losing 1pound a week but not tracking your food intake and eating a lot of sugar outside the anabolic window then you are not going to complete the task.

Use a wingman

I bet you thought I was going to say find Goose from *Top Gun* or some other friend to go to the gym with you right? If you can find someone who will truly help you, then great but the third and, in my opinion, most powerful tactic to battling hunger is actually to use supplements such as protein powder.

Not nearly as cool as Goose I know, but unlike Goose, protein supplements don't die. They also make excellent dependable wingmen. The reason they are so powerful a tool in battling hunger is they make the other two tactics MUCH easier to execute. They allow us to easily get more protein and fats into our food plan at the expense of carbohydrates and they help us ensure we do not end up in a large energy deficit.

An average high-quality protein shake contains 25 grams of protein and only 2 grams of carbs and 2 grams of fat. To get that much protein you would have to eat 4 whole eggs and you would also get 12 grams of fat along with them.

If you are concerned that protein supplements are expensive, think again. A serving of high-quality whey protein powder, such as the highly popular Optimum Nutrition, is 78 cents. The same amount of protein in raw eggs cost approximately 67 cents. Unless you are eating your eggs raw, you still have to cook them. Plus I keep a bin of protein powder in the trunk of my car, which is extremely convenient.

It is also hard to eat your body weight in grams of protein every day even if you are focused on it. A 200-pound man would need to eat five meals a day each containing 40 grams of protein. That is basically one chicken breast every meal for five meals. On the other hand, I can prepare and drink a protein shake in less than two minutes and get the same amount of protein with very little carbs or fats. That means I get to eat those carbs and fats as real food. And by the way, modern shakes are delicious. If you don't like one brand or flavor of shake you will definitely find one that you do like. My favorite flavor is banana cream. I also like to mix orange creatine with vanilla protein. It tastes like a Dreamsicle.

If that same 200-lb man got three servings of protein from shakes a day, he would only have to eat 125 grams of protein. That is doable. A 130 lb. woman could drink two servings of protein a day and only have to eat 75 grams of protein. That is 25 grams over three meals, which is not that difficult. Unless you have prepared all your meals beforehand, I would say that most modern lifestyles make it extremely difficult to prepare and eat 5-6 meals a day. The shakes make this food plan possible for our busy lifestyles.

Using protein supplements allows us to better execute the first tactic against hunger: get more protein and good fats into our food plan at the expense of carbohydrates. If we need more fats we can just add coconut oil, flaxseed oil, peanut butter, almond butter, or some other healthy fat into the shake. If we need more carbs we can add healthy oats or fruit to also get micronutrients and very important fiber.

Using shakes also allows us to more easily accomplish the second tactic against hunger: don't end up in a large caloric deficit. If I realize at the end of the day that I didn't eat enough, I can quickly and easily make a protein shake that contains the necessary amount of protein, fat, and carbs. Protein supplements allow us to eat five to six meals in a day. Yes, natural food is preferred, but I can't prepare and consume five to six meals every day. I would rather focus on my workouts or spending time with my family.

Protein shakes are fast, convenient, and effective. You can reach your goals without supplements but it is much more difficult. If you are truly against supplements I recommend you research the evidence for and against them for yourself. Protein powder and creatine have been thoroughly tested over the 20 years they have been used by athletes around the world. There is little to no evidence that either of these products has any negative impact, while countless studies demonstrate their effectiveness in creating more muscle and losing more fat than not using them. If you're not cheating, you're not trying. The bottom line is that supplements give us a huge advantage in maintaining a food plan.

Avoiding and suppressing unhealthy SAM threats

My family and I have been lucky enough to be stationed in Korea, Italy, Alaska, Turkey, and Phoenix. There was delicious food in all of those locations, but Italy and Turkey were the obvious highlights. If you don't like kimchi, Korean food is not going to please you that much. If you can kill it yourself, Alaskan food is delicious but otherwise only the Thai food is decent (at least in Central/Northern Alaska). But to my mind, the Mediterranean diet is by far the healthiest and most delicious.

After living overseas for almost 10 years, coming back to American food was an eye-opener. My first impression was that it was also delicious. My second impression was that it was extremely dense and there was a ton of sugar in everything. There was also a lot of it. No other culture I have been in has the doggy bag. We get more food than we can eat in one sitting, so we package up the rest and carry it home. The plates and the portion sizes are just huge in this country.

Even if the calories are counted incorrectly with the antiquated Atwater system, American food just has too much energy in it. Not once in Korea or Turkey did I feel overly full. As a kid growing up in the U.S., I remember walking out of restaurants with difficulty because my stomach was so full. This is not what we want in an age where food is readily available. Back when we were hunting the woolly mammoth and needed to replenish 5% of our body weight after an exhaustive hunt, we needed to over-consume. More recently, before WWII, most working Americans engaged in manual labor, like farming for example, but today most Americans work in office or service jobs and sit most of the day.[15] When we over-consume in today's world, we just get fat.

We put sugar in everything. Try and not eat sugar or processed carbs at a restaurant in America, it is virtually impossible. Even the Korean, Italian, and Turkish restaurants in the US add a lot of sugar to their food. The Korean restaurants give you much

---

[15] Marlene A. Lee and Mark Mather, "U.S. Labor Force Trends," *Population Bulletin* 63, no. 2 (2008): 9; http://www.prb.org/pdf08/63.2uslabor.pdf.

more rice and the sauces all have sugar in them. In Korea, there was often no rice on the table. It was normally weird roots, strange pickled vegetables, or some crazy sea creature. In Korean culture they say overweight people "eat too much rice."

The drinks are giant in the US and with free refills, they're also unending. This is also an American novelty and completely foreign to the cultures I have witnessed. If you look around and wonder why there are so many overweight people in the US, just look at an average dinner in a chain restaurant. Even kids' meals are giant. One normal kids' meal has enough carbs and fats to recharge me after a strenuous leg workout. My stomach will also probably hurt.

We need to think of US restaurants and parties as known SAM threats. In order to ensure we hit the primary targets and give ourselves the best opportunity to see motivating results by hitting the secondary target, we need to avoid or suppress the temptation of restaurant and party food. As I explained earlier, the best tactic is to avoid a SAM. If we keep the unhealthy food out of our sight and smell range we are completely safe, but this is not a viable long-term tactic. We still want to enjoy life and hang out with friends and family at restaurants and parties. This is where protein supplements and a little prior planning can greatly increase our defenses.

In combat against real SAM systems, we always want to first learn the most intel we can on the SAM's location and capability. In the planning phase we ensure that our SAM suppression air assets are in front of the strike package to shoot radar-seeking missiles at the SAMs and use electronic attack. All strike aircraft also turn on and check their electronic self-defense systems. We fly outside of the SAM ring if we can. If we have to enter the SAM's threat ring we have our radar-defeating chaff ready. If we get SAM tracking indications in our radar warning receivers, at that point we are ready to start our aggressive maneuvers to defeat the radar and the missile.

Facing a dietary SAM you should follow the same process. Plan to avoid the SAM if possible. First off, don't buy unhealthy food from the grocery store. Don't live at home with a dietary SAM. Don't shop hungry. Drink a protein shake before you go to the grocery store or make a list while you are not hungry. Buy vegetables, fruits, and whole foods. Buy your food whole and fresh, not in boxes (unless inside the box is whole fresh food). Stay away from the middle of the grocery store. Don't worry so much about fat, just try and keep the food fresh and avoid the fast-digesting carbs.

Second, try and avoid the unhealthy SAM restaurants. If you don't feel good after the meal or feel bloated leaving the restaurant, then chances are it was an unhealthy restaurant. Or maybe you just ordered the wrong food, but unfortunately some places don't even have one good healthy option. Unlimited bread sticks at Olive Garden? Worst idea ever. Even the salads come loaded with processed croutons and sugar in the dressings. If you can avoid the threat and go somewhere else or cook a healthy meal at home, in the long run you will reach your goals much faster.

If you can't avoid the threat then your only option is to suppress it. I believe the best technique is to eat a healthy meal or drink a protein shake before going to the restaurant or party. The pre-party shake is like the fighter pilot's electronic self-defense system. We make ourselves harder to detect. The wimpy voice is silenced by the shake. We don't have to rely on willpower to keep ourselves safe from the threat. American party food is lethal. It's delicious and unhealthy. Most of the time at a party there is no healthy option. If I am not hungry when I show up I can suppress the wimpy voice and still enjoy the delicious unhealthy food. Our skinny chef friend in Italy ate pasta every day, but like she said, "I don't eat an entire bowl..."

I can eat a moderate amount of fast-digesting carbs at a party but it doesn't become my main meal. I already drank my main meal before I arrived and it contained no carbs or fat so I can eat some carbs and fat at the party without hurting my overall food plan. This is how supplements help us plan the unhealthy food into our food plans. They supplement it.

Cheat to win

The final tactic we will employ is the cheat day. I explained before about blind spots in our understanding of basic biochemistry. Many processes in the body are still not well understood by modern science. The body is an extremely complex, organic machine made up of literally trillions of living cells. That is a lot of moving parts. We can't just stop adding a particular fuel to the body and expect it not to react.

By lowering carbs and calories at the same time we run the risk of forcing the body into starvation mode. We have to coax the fat off the body by convincing it that all is well and that there is no food shortage. It can comfortably give up its energy reserves and everything will be okay. We can help convince the body of this by allowing it to eat whatever it wants one day a week.

One day a week you can eat literally *whatever you want*. I know this sounds crazy but it is actually a very powerful tool in this food plan for a few reasons. First, it replenishes carbs and in body building circles is often called a re-feed day or a balance day. This keeps the body from hanging on to its fat reserves. Second, it gives us more motivation to stick to our food plan on the six other days because we know we will be able to eat whatever we want on our cheat day. As Baumeister and Tierney explain in *Willpower: Rediscovering the Greatest Human Strength*, it is much harder to deliver an indefinite "no" to the brain than it is to say, "later." It is easier to tell ourselves we will just eat it later in the week on our cheat day than to just never eat the food. We are able to suppress the threat until a different day when maybe, we won't want the food at all.

The third benefit of a cheat day is that it keeps our morale high and allows us to maintain our motivation in the long term. Eating just broccoli and chicken breasts every day gets old fast (unless those happen to be your favorite foods). Eating pizza, cake, and ice cream is a true joy of life and I don't want to give them up, especially when I don't have to in order to reach my goals.

We want our food plan to be livable and long term. You don't have to give up on your favorite sugary foods. Simply don't eat them all the time. Save them to eat within 60 minutes after your workouts or your cheat day. A cheat day not only allows us to maintain our food plan in the long term, but it can actually help us by re-feeding the body and coaxing it to give up fat more easily on the other six days.

If you still aren't on board with the cheat meal idea, think about this. Eating unhealthy foods one day a week will not make you fat, just as eating healthy foods one day a week will not make you skinny. If you eat pizza, chicken wings, and ice cream over your daily caloric limit six days a week, but don't eat anything on the seventh day you will still most likely gain fat. Six out of seven days you are eating unhealthy. That is 86% of the time. But if you eat healthy 86% of the time I promise you will reach your goals. That is *most* of the time. If you eat healthy food that has roughly a third of each macronutrient, with fiber and low amounts of fast-digesting carbs, you have a winning and doable long-term food plan. There is no option but for your body to change. It is simple math.

Having that one cheat day will give our brains the motivation to stay on this food plan and it will give our body reason to give up its fat. Having cheat days also allows us to go to normal events with friends and family and still participate. We can eat and drink whatever we want on a Friday night out. We can eat the cake and drink the coke at a birthday party. It is not a big deal at all and it fits into our food plan. Just make the day of that event your cheat day for the week. Then the other six days, eat as healthy as you can. If you find yourself craving something, just tell yourself you can eat it on your cheat day and eat something healthier instead. Just think long term and make gradual changes. Objectively observe your food intake, your weight, and your workout performance. Decide each week to continue or to change it up slightly. Then act on your decision. Get inside your own body's OODA loop. The canyon will start to form. Once the habits are in place, it is no longer a food plan, it is just how you eat.

Conclusion

We're All Gonna Die

I listened to a man on a TV show recount how he learned of his stage 4 terminal lung cancer. The doctor said he had six months to live. He went home, curled up in a ball, and cried himself to sleep. After a week of crying he decided to finally fulfill his long-term dream to build a house in the mountains. The show then showed him in front of his newly built mountain house looking extremely happy. He was throwing a Frisbee with his wife and daughter.

"Why didn't he just build the damn house sooner?" I thought. He looks ridiculously happy and the man has stage 4 terminal lung cancer. Imagine if he was completely healthy.

I bring this up because we are all six months from dying. You could die right now reading this sentence. Literally. One of those trillion cells in your body could mess up, start a blood clot, and bam, brain-dead. It happens all the time.

In Iraq, time and again, we were jolted awake from the dead of sleep by the mortars or louder and more terrifying explosive ordinance detonations. I would lie on the ground imagining a mortar flying right into the bunk for hours. The odds were low but it happened to a few other bunks when we were there. It was scary and it was tough to get back to sleep.

After a while I think we just got tired of being scared to die. I'm still scared to die, but I'm just tired of being scared of it. It is going to happen and it could honestly happen tomorrow. I try and live my life as if it's going to end in six months because all of us, just like the happy man up in the mountains, are going to die. You are going to die. We're all gonna die.

Do you think you are going to look back from your deathbed and say "yeah, I had an easy life…it was great but I wish I had watched more TV and drunk more beer…"? Screw that. I want to go down having made a positive impact on this world. The first place you start making a positive impact is on your own body. The mind will follow. I believe the program I outlined in this book is powerful because it is sustainable in the long term. If you make this program a priority and apply the OODA loop process to hit the targets, you will ultimately and without a doubt succeed. Millions of other people have done it. It is completely doable.

But these days, everyone wants an easy workout program. It's not about easy, it's about sustainable. They want to just follow a program and not put any thought or effort into it. Then they are amazed when it doesn't work. Well no shit it didn't work, from the very beginning all you wanted was an easy program with no effort.

What in life comes without having to do anything hard? It might be hard, fine. Sometimes it's hard, get over it. And sometime you are going to die, get over it. Do you want to die having done nothing difficult in your life? Or do you want to have made a positive impact on yourself and the world around you?

If you liked this book and want to receive updates on my future books as well as free guides, join my readers list at www.chrislehto.com. I honestly wish the best for you. If you read this entire book, then you obviously want to improve. If you don't use my program then find something else that you will use. Just don't quit, stay on target.

Made in the USA
San Bernardino, CA
02 March 2017